Keto Diet

How to Use the Ketogenic Diet to Lose Weight, Burn Fat, and Increase Mental Clarity, Including How to Get into Ketosis and Fasting on Keto for Beginners

Contents

Introduction

The following chapters will discuss how you can easily and smoothly transition from your regular diet to the keto diet, a diet that is driven by eating low-carbs and high fats. It has a ton of benefits, including weight loss, more energy, better workouts, and a sharper and better focus. No matter what your reasons are for checking out the keto diet, you will find these in here and more.

This book will go over more than just the science and the idea of the keto diet. It will also go into the benefits, myths, truths, exercising on a diet, what the keto flu is and how to deal with it, and a whole bunch of other information you might need.

The idea of this book is not to list a whole bunch of recipes and tell you just to eat this; you will work this out. There is nobody here telling you what you should be eating and when you should be eating. The idea is to give you the information you need to help yourself start to find the foods you like and cook the way you want to cook. This book will help you put together a meal plan that you will love, and look forward to cooking.

Chapter 1: The Beginning

How does the keto diet work, and why is it so different from other diets?

The keto diet is when you train your body to use primarily the fats that you eat for energy. You take control of your metabolism that way, putting in motion a process called Ketosis. Ketosis uses the fats that you consume to create the energy your body needs.

That's the short explanation. Here's the long one:

In the basic sense, the keto diet is typically one of low carbs, moderate protein, and high fats. This causes the body to produce what are called ketones. Now, because you probably don't know what "ketones" means, here is a list of vocabulary you should know before you get started. It will make things easier to understand for later on.

Ketones: The chemicals that emerge and multiply once you start burning fat for energy. They are converted from stored body fat in the liver. The more you eat more fat and fewer carbs, the more your body will produce them.

Carbs: Also known as carbohydrates, carbs are molecules that contain carbon, hydrogen, and oxygen atoms. They are also one of the three macronutrients. The other two are fat and protein.

Glucose: You might be more familiar with its other name, blood sugar. Glucose is the chemical that is the easiest to break down in the body, making it an easy source of energy. Glucose gets converted into glycogen, which is stored for energy use. Excess glucose gets converted into fat stores.

Insulin: A hormone made in the pancreas. Insulin is what the body needs to break down sugar, or glucose, or carbs. Insulin is necessary for your body, as it is used to help keep your blood sugar from getting too high or too low. Diabetes is when your pancreas can no longer create insulin.

Carbs are often considered what the body needs for energy. Glucose is the easiest form of sugar that the body can break down, and the easiest form of energy it can use. However, if you deprive your body of carbs or glucose, you can make it burn fat for energy instead. When you burn fat for energy instead of carbs, your body enters what is called "Ketosis". Ergo, the Keto Diet.

When you eat fat and carbs, your body automatically starts to use the carbs as its main source of energy. This is because carbs are easy to break down into glucose and be used for energy. When your body uses glucose for energy, your fat energy automatically gets stored to be used later by insulin. It becomes difficult to burn that stored fat because you're always refilling your bloodstream with more glucose.

Your body will always go for the easiest way to fuel you, regardless of what other fuel you're giving it. By reducing carbs, and instead of feeding your body fats, you're taking control of what energy you want your body to be using. You're forcing your body to switch to burning fats rather than carbs after it starves itself of glucose.

Carbs are often hailed as the best kind of fuel for your body, but that isn't true. You can only store about 2,500 calories worth of carbs in your body. But you can store up to 30,000 calories worth of fat! That is a huge amount of energy, and imagine the number of things you can do with it.

When your body makes the switch, you'll be putting it into a state of Ketosis. You've probably already been in a state of Ketosis after not eating for a few hours, like when you sleep. Ketosis is the state of when your body makes the transition from burning glucose to burning your fat cells. You start to make ketones after about 12 hours of not having any sugar or carbs. This effectively puts your body into a state of Ketosis.

It a completely natural metabolic process when the body does not have enough glucose for energy, leading it to burn fat in its place. Very simple, very natural, and very good for you. It can take a while for your body to get used to this, but eventually, you'll end up feeling so much better because of it.

Types of Keto Diets

There are several different types of keto diets. This book will mostly refer to the standard keto diet. However, there are options out there, and it's about choosing the right option for you. All of these diets can help you lose weight, burn fat, and balance blood sugar levels. All of them have their benefits and objectives. It's really all about what you want. Here is a comprehensive list of all of them to help you figure out which one will work for you:

Standard Ketogenic Diet

The standard ketogenic diet is best for beginners. It's also good for anyone looking into losing body fat and those who suffer from insulin resistance. Daily macros would look like this:

Protein Intake: 0.8 grams per pound of lean body mass, adequate

Carb Intake: 20 to 50 every day, 5% total calories, low

Fat Intake: 70% to 75% of total calories

Anyone who is just starting out with the keto diet should stick to this one before looking into other options. You might find yourself struggling with just how restrictive the diet is and will want to get used to Ketosis before switching over. Even then, you should only switch over if you feel like it's the right choice for you.

High-Protein Ketogenic Diet

If your goal is to build extra muscle and you've already tried and enjoyed the effects of the keto diet, consider this one. It's great for bodybuilders, weightlifters, and athletes—the people who need larger amounts of protein in their diet and need to build more muscle and get stronger. This is what their daily macros would look like:

Protein Intake: 35% of calories

Carb Intake: 5% of calories

Fat Intake: 60% of calories

Cyclical Ketogenic Diet

The cyclical ketogenic diet involves eating keto and low carbs for five to six days out of the week and then spending that remaining one or two days eating a high amount of carbs. It's good for bodybuilders and other athletes to maximize fat loss while building lean mass. Don't pick this one if you find yourself needing a bit of a break. It doesn't permit you to eat as much chocolate as you'd like. You still have to be eating healthy carbs.

Five to Six Days Keto Macros:

Protein Intake: 20% to 25% of calories

Carb Intakes: 5% of calories

Fat Intake: 70% to 75% of calories

Two to One Day Carb-Loading Macros:

Protein Intake: 20% to 25% of calories

Carb Intake: 70% of calories

Fat Intake: 5% to 10% of calories

Targeted Ketogenic Diet

The targeted ketogenic diet is where you target carb consumption around your workouts, a hybrid between the standard keto diet and the cyclical keto diet. It allows you to train at higher intensities at the gym and is a great option for people who are looking to maintain a high exercise performance. You eat on a regular keto diet the majority of the time, but all of your carbs are eating around your workout. Usually, about 20 to 50 grams total, before and after.

If you're already on a typical keto diet, it might be worth it to make the switch if you're looking to build up some muscle or if you find yourself struggling with your workout routine.

There is no straightforward answer for what kind of keto diet you should be on. Everyone is different. When you're just starting off, you should be trying different things, keeping track of what works and what doesn't, and paying attention to your body. Keeping track of things in something like a fitness app will help.

The Truth about Carbs

Carbs have gotten a very bad rap in these modern diet times. You're told, over and over again, that you must stop eating carbs if you ever want to lose weight, get healthier, or look better. Or you can't eat them unless you work out, or keep them contained in one meal, etc. Well, in rebuttal to this, anyone who follows a keto diet correctly understands that carbs are a must in any healthy diet, even if it's just a little bit.

Carbs are actually needed in your diet. They're one of the three essential macronutrients, along with protein and fat. So, what's the problem?

Well, we eat too many of them. Plus, most of the carbs we do eat come from unhealthy sources, such as fast food, starchy vegetables, and huge serving sizes. Too many carbs affect your blood sugar dramatically, leading to a risk of diabetes, constipation, atherosclerosis (a condition that causes disruptions in the bloodstream, leading to heart attacks) and vascular diseases. The biggest issue with carbs isn't the fact that we eat them; we eat too many of them, and when we do, they're not the carbs we should be eating.

This is why even if you decide that the keto diet isn't right for you, seriously consider looking at the number of carbs you are consuming. If your goal is to lose weight, remember: any carbs that are not needed by your body are automatically stored as body fat.

What Makes Us Fat

It is somewhat weird. It's called fat, but it doesn't make us fat. This made sense years ago when we just assumed that the fat in our food was causing the fat around our middles. It just added up. This started the whole "no fat added" campaign, which didn't help. If something says "low fat," this is basically just a label saying "there is a ton of refined sugar and carbs in this." So, stay away!

Healthy fats, such as what is in avocados, olive oil, and nuts, actually help you. They work to process all the food we're putting into our bodies, and our brains are actually 60% fat, so it's good for it too. Fats are very complex (which is why there is an entire chapter in this book devoted to them).

So what does make us fat? Well, this goes back to the sugar and carbs. If you eat more than what you need, they will be transformed into fat cells and put into "storage". This is the same with any food you eat. If you eat more than what you need, or over your calorie quota, you will gain weight. That's just how it is.

Mythbusting with the Keto Diet

The keto diet has gotten a lot of flak in the past few years. Many people have brushed it aside, assuming that it's just another fad diet. Of course, we know by now that it's not and that it will be around for years yet as a great way to lose weight and get your health back on track.

The Keto diet has numerous misconceptions and myths surrounding it, some of which you may have bought into. You should never go into a diet not knowing what is true, and what isn't true. You need to be well informed with the solid facts. Here are some of them, and the truth:

Myth 1: You can eat as much fat as you want, and it doesn't matter what kind you fill your plate with.

As much as we all wish there were a diet out there where you could pile your plate full of bacon and cheese without having to worry, the keto diet is not it. Until science gets there, we can just dream, and be realistic. No, **the keto diet's focus is on unsaturated fats**. Foods full of heart-and-blood healthy unsaturated fats such as avocados, nuts, olive oil, and fish, rather than saturated fats like cake, cooking margarine, and fatty cuts of meat like beef and pork. Even if all you're eating are unsaturated fats, you should be sticking to calorie counting and serving sizes. Calories are still calories, and too many will make you gain weight.

Myth 2: You can go on and off it no problem. It's a temporary thing, and you don't have to worry about gaining the weight back. It will stay off without any effort. Nope. Inconsistency with the keto diet will not just make you gain all the weight back; you won't experience the full value of Ketosis.

There have been reports of people who just do it for a few weeks before going back to their original diet, or even less time. This won't keep your weight off, and you will have an even harder time reaching that state of Ketosis.

Myth 3: The Keto diet is high on protein.

The Keto diet is not a high protein diet. **Protein should be eaten in moderation and kept careful track of using a scale**. Excess protein is converted into glucose which spikes your blood sugar. It also can lead to increased ketones, which sounds good, but can be problematic if you already have a high level in your body. Every person's protein intake is different and takes many things into consideration, such as exercise level, weight, sex, and age. If you're an athlete, for example, you'll need a higher protein intake than someone who only exercises moderately.

Myth 4: The amount of carbs a person needs is always the same, no matter the person.

People make the mistake of not knowing how many carbs are involved in a keto diet, or they don't understand just how little carbs it requires. On average, it's only about 20 to 50 grams of carbohydrates a day, which really isn't very much. To put that in perspective, a cup of spaghetti, cooked, without any added salt, is 43.3 grams of carbs. A medium apple, fresh with skin, is about 19 grams of carbs. The amount of carbs that you need during the day depends on the person. **Depending on your lifestyle, you may be able to go higher**. If you're unsure, make an appointment with a dietician or nutritionist who will be able to help you calculate what you need.

Myth 5: Veggies and fruit are high in carbs. You can't eat them.

Only do this if you have a desire for constipation, which can be a nasty keto side effect. **You need fiber**, and veggies and fruits are some of the best sources of it. They also have a ton of vitamins and minerals and antioxidants that are great for your body. The reality is: there are not a whole lot of food types out there that are completely free of carbs. You'll be hard pressed to find them, and the only things that will be completely carb free are oils, butter, and meats. Stick to veggies that aren't starchy (think potatoes and yams), and vegetables like broccoli, spinach, cauliflower, and zucchini. If you need sweetness, go for berries like raspberries and blueberries. There are plenty of awesome ways to make these ingredients delicious.

Myth 6: When you go on the keto diet, your body goes into ketoacidosis.

Ketoacidosis refers to diabetic ketoacidosis and is a condition related to Type 1 diabetes. People often get this and **Ketosis, the state that your body goes into when you go on the keto diet**, mixed up. Ketoacidosis is life-threatening, can develop in as little as 24 hours, and occurs when the body does not get enough insulin. Often when people hear the word "Ketosis", they immediately think "ketoacidosis". If people ask, be sure to explain the difference.

Myth 7: The keto diet by itself will help you lose weight.

People often go on the keto diet for this reason. Maybe it's the reason you picked up this book. The reality is: **there is no such thing as a diet that will automatically work for everyone**. Success in losing weight, and putting your health back on track, can and probably will be a long journey. It involves being consistent with an eating plan. People have different blood sugar responses to different foods. To figure out an eating plan that will work for you, please visit a nutritionist or dietician.

Why Should You Do the Keto Diet

The keto diet is great for weight loss, but it also has a host of other benefits. When you run your body on fats rather than carbs, your blood sugar will be more stable. You'll have a lower risk of diseases like heart problems and Type 2 diabetes. It will help cool inflammation in your body and reverse conditions such as a fatty liver and Metabolic Syndrome (a cluster of conditions: increased blood pressure, high blood sugar, excess body fat around the waist). Overall, you'll feel better.

Now, the question really is: should you do the keto diet? The keto diet will only work the way you want it to work for certain people. It all depends on your body. Genetics, body weight, age, gender— these things can all have an impact on your results.

The truth is that in the days of the cavemen, our diet would've been similar to a keto one. Lots of veggies, protein, and very few carbs— mostly because a lot of the carbs we eat today didn't exist. Our focus would've been on food that we needed to keep us healthy and full and strong, not on foods that would send our blood sugars spiking.

You should also keep in mind that some people should not do the keto diet for health reasons, as they might have a condition that will only worsen if they do, and it could be catastrophic for their health. This is why you should always check with a doctor before you embark on any big change in your diet, keto or otherwise. You should not try the keto diet if you have one of the following conditions:

- Carnitine deficiency (primary)
- Carnitine palmitoyltransferase (CPT) I or II deficiency
- Carnitine translocase deficiency
- Beta-oxidation defects
- Mitochondrial 3-hydroxy-3-methylglutaryl-CoA synthase (mHMGS) deficiency
- Medium-chain acyl dehydrogenase deficiency (MCAD)
- Long-chain acyl dehydrogenase deficiency (LCAD)
- Short-chain acyl dehydrogenase deficiency (SCAD)
- Long-chain 3-hydroxyacyl-CoA deficiency
- Medium-chain 3-hydroxyacyl-CoA deficiency
- Pyruvate carboxylase deficiency
- Porphyria

If you have any of these conditions, except for porphyria, they are usually identified early on in someone's life. Porphyria can be identified later on. If you have one of these conditions, you'll likely already know. However, you still should check with your doctor.

You should also ask your doctor's advice on the keto diet if your medical history, including your family history, includes any of the following conditions:

- Kidney Failure

- Pancreatitis

- Abdominal Tumors

- Gastric Bypass Surgery

- Gallbladder Disease

- Poor Nutritional Status

- Impaired Liver Function

- Impaired Fat Digestion

- Pregnancy and/or lactation

Keep in mind that doctors are not trained in nutrition all that much. They're not experts on the subject. They're often taught that Ketosis is dangerous, and thus don't know all that much about it. In fact, many doctors might very well get "Ketosis" confused with "ketoacidosis". If you want to make sure that they know this distinction, take this book to show them.

It is because of this that you should really consider seeing a trained nutritionist or dietician. They're specifically taught to figure out what people should eat and can explain to you what effect different foods will have on your body. A good one will be able to walk you through everything you need to know and tailor something specifically for your body. They will also likely know all about Ketosis and have easy plans on how to get you into it. There is a handy guide below if you do plan on visiting one.

Also, one last thing to keep in mind: a keto diet must be done right, no exceptions. In this book, we'll be taking you through every step of the way. So don't let yourself worry about whether or not you're messing up. You got this.

Common Mistakes Keto Beginners Make

We all make mistakes. It's part of life. However, avoiding them is a much more preferred option, especially when it comes to things like your body and its health. Thankfully, the keto diet, despite being new, encompasses many people who have made the below mistakes and now you can learn from them. Read this list, and hopefully, you can avoid the derailments of your ketogenic journey.

Obsessing over your scale. If you're in this to gain weight, it can be easy to get attached to the number on the scale. You weigh yourself several times a day, you have the number written down in several different places, and you always have the number of pounds you have lost memorized.

The keto diet has a lot of great benefits, and one of these benefits is weight loss. People have reported losing up to ten pounds in their first *week*. This isn't what you should be focusing on, even if your goal is to lose weight. For one, scale numbers rarely give the whole picture. There will be a ton of progress that doesn't even show up on the scale (also keep in mind that if you're working out, you'll be gaining muscle, which weighs more than fat). If you really want to measure your progress, consider buying a cheap measuring tape for sewing (you can get them very inexpensively at dollar stores), and use that instead. This will tell you much more about what is happening to your body than your scale ever would, and you'll see the progress happening right before your very eyes.

Also, two, the number can make you feel as if you're not doing well. It can make you feel as if you're not improving at all, even if you are, and might have you feeling discouraged. Keeping track of your journey is great, but how about focusing on how great you feel? Focus on how you can walk up the stairs without getting winded and how your skin has never been so clear? These things might keep you more motivated than a stupid number ever could.

Not enough fats. The average person is not used to their diet being 70% fats. They often underestimate just how much it is, and just how many you need to consume in a day to enter Ketosis. If you're 140 pounds, and you want to maintain your weight, you'd be eating about 160 grams of fat per day. To put that into perspective, an avocado is about 30 grams of fat per one whole fruit. To get 160 grams of fat, you'd be eating about five and a half avocados per day. Crazy, right? (Also, to be clear, these numbers are very rough so please don't take them at face value. Please do your own macro measurements for your body and lifestyle.)

If you want to make sure you're getting enough fats, be sure to track things like macros and use an app to figure out where you can get more of the good stuff.

Not eating good fats. People often get saturated fats and unsaturated fats confused. The whole "no fat added" and "fat-free" epidemic has done nothing to help that. If you're eating all the bad fats all day (think anything with trans fats), you're not going to reach Ketosis. If you're getting all these good and healthy fats, like nuts, olive oil, and fish, you'll definitely benefit.

As long as you stick to foods that you know are real and wholesome, with nothing added that you don't know what it is, you should find yourself entering Ketosis. Just avoid anything that has the words "fat-free" on it.

Too much protein. This is a very common mistake for beginner ketogenic dieters. When entering Ketosis, or keeping your body in Ketosis, you only need a moderate amount of protein because your body is using fats for energy. You only really need protein for building and maintaining muscle mass, so you will probably find yourself needing much less than you expect.

Keep in mind that if you eat too much protein, especially too often, the protein in your body will go through a process called gluconeogenesis, a process where other nutrients other than carbs convert into glucose. This will knock you out of Ketosis, and you'll have to start over. This process is pretty slow, so you don't have to worry too much about it, but it's just something to remember—another good reminder as to why it's important to track macros.

Not meal planning. This is the biggest mistake that beginner dieters make. They assume that because they have the idea in their mind, they can just stay on track. Think of meal planning almost like a map that is telling you directly where to go. By planning and making your meals in advance, you're removing temptation that could throw you out of Ketosis and helping yourself avoid falling short of your daily macro needs. By meal planning, you're literally giving yourself all the options you need without any need to order food. This can also help you maintain what is working and discard what is not. Plus, it saves time that is spent in the kitchen. You also might be able to find some amazing meals out there that you never would've tried before!

If you're not into cooking at all, well, you're going to have a hard time with the keto diet unless you have a private chef. Get into cooking by keeping it simple. Just focus on nailing these daily macros and then you can figure out how to put grill marks on the chicken.

Looking for a quick fix. One of the worst things that modern advertising and branding have done for living a healthy lifestyle is constantly referring to them as "diets". Diets imply something temporary. It implies that once it's over, you can go back to doing the same kind of eating you were doing before. The keto diet, and any brand of healthy living, such as the Atkins diet, veganism, or going gluten-free, is a lifestyle. It's not something you can switch on for a few months then switch off. You'll just find yourself right back where you started.

You might find yourself getting on the keto diet, and get yourself obsessed. You're obsessed with the results, you're obsessed with how great you look and feel, and you're obsessed with how trim your waistline is. You keep at it because it feels awesome to be healthy and to live your best life. Others, on the other hand, may reach that magic number on the scale or the tape measure and figure that they're done. They don't need to measure calories anymore or focus on the ratio of carbs, fats, and protein in their diet. However, they always wind up where they started—addicted to sugar and bad carbs and struggling to wean themselves off them.

If you're just looking to drop some pounds and that's all you want, consider just removing sugar entirely from your diet. It will cause a healthy drop in weight, and as long as you stick to it, the weight will stay off.

Not Getting Enough Sleep. You need sleep. Seven to eight hours of it, preferably. Lack of sleep can cause slip-ups, and make you crave bad foods. It also makes you hungrier, and it's harder for you to stop eating. You crave unhealthy food and want nothing more than to dive right into a basket of fries for that quick sugar rush to get yourself through the day until bed. Sleep is critical to your mental and physical health, so get yourself enough of it.

Not Drinking Enough Water. Your body needs water. In adult men, it makes up about 60% of the body. In adult women, it makes up about 55%. Either way, that's more than half. Water flushes out toxins, regulates body temperature, and improves digestion. You need water, especially if before you got all of your liquids from carb loaded drinks, like soft drinks, orange juice, and vitamin water. If you really dislike the plain taste of water, consider adding slices of lemon. However, the taste does grow on you after a while.

Comparing Yourself to Other People. This goes hand in hand with not focusing too much on the scale. Yes, the keto diet does lead to weight loss, an easier time focusing and feeling better about life overall, but you might find yourself wondering why you aren't getting these same results as fast as others. Every person's body is different, in both big and small ways. Comparing yourself to others also leads to big insecurities on whether or not you're doing the right thing.

On the keto diet, there are often very similar outcomes; they just happen at different paces. Don't focus on everyone else's results. Focus on yours, and how great you're doing. Everything should be done at your pace, and everybody's journey is different.

Doing it alone. Nobody should ever have to do something completely alone. Having people help you on your journey, and give you the support that you want, cannot be replaced by anything. It's a great feeling knowing that people want this for you, just as much as you want this for you. Doing things by yourself is difficult. So let your friends and family know about this lifestyle change you are embarking on. You don't want them tempting you by offering food that the Ketosis diet can't support. Maybe one or two may want to join you on your journey! But let your friends and family know. There's a whole bunch of ideas and tips on how to build this support system in this book!

Visiting a Dietician (or a Nutritionist)

Taking the step of going and visiting a dietician is a big step. While visiting any doctor can be nerve-wracking, visiting a dietician can make someone especially nervous. After all, the definition of a dietician is someone who looks at your current diet and tells you what you should be changing. Yeah, not fun. We have a hard time telling our family doctor everything that's up (which is not a good thing, stop doing that), so it's even harder visiting someone we probably have never met before, and just telling them everything. It can be a great experience, though, where you learn about your body and what it needs to be healthy.

Visiting a dietician is a great way of educating yourself. With a dietician, you can figure out what you need to eat, when you need to eat, find new recipes, and learn about all the benefits that come with your diet. You can clarify ahead that you're interested in trying a keto diet, and they'll have a host of information for you right at their fingertips. They can be a great motivator and partner for you in this journey.

Visiting a dietician should not be a painful experience. It should be one of enlightenment, and you should walk out feeling like someone really just helped you. It can be a great experience working with a dietician. Keep that in mind as you go in. Here are some tips on how to approach it, and what you can do to make the process easier:

- Be open-minded and positive. Walking into their office, make sure you know that they might say some things you won't enjoy hearing. Like you are eating too many bad fats, or you're not getting enough fiber intake. They might give you some hard truths. Look on the bright side, and open your mind up to the idea that they are only telling you this because they want to help you.

- Don't lie! Many people feel embarrassed about their eating habits. You need to work past any shame you have because the only way a dietician can help you is if they know what you're putting into your body. Don't claim that you eat salads three times a week when, really, it's more like three times a year. A dietician is not there to judge you; they're there to help you.

- Keep a food journal for a few weeks leading up to it. Leading up to your meeting, for at least a week, keep an honest food journal. Don't lie. Again, do not lie. Make a note of everything you eat. This will be helpful to act as a roadmap for the dietician, telling exactly where you need to go and what you need to change.

- Have a list of any medication or supplements you are taking. If you're on any medications, whether they're prescribed or not, let them know. If you have any long-term or permanent conditions, like diabetes, let them know. It could affect your diet.

- Consider a list of foods that you like. Really love chocolate? Put it on the list. Love carrots but would rather eat a shoe than broccoli? Put it on the list. This way your dietitian will be able to help you find recipes that they know you will like. They want to make eating a fun and interesting experience for you, not a chore. They don't want to fill your plate with foods you're going to hate eating.

• Understand that there is no such thing as one diet that works for everyone. Yes, we know that you're interested in the keto diet, but it may not be the one for you, thanks to health reasons. Or maybe your lifestyle. The keto diet doesn't always work for everyone, and that's OKAY. We're all different. That doesn't mean you shouldn't try, but just be aware that it may not work. Our society needs to drop this idea of there being one diet out there for the entire world. No. Everybody has different needs and will respond differently to different foods.

• Be clear about what goals you have. Go in knowing what you want. Is it to lose weight? Is it to look better? Is it to get healthier? Is it to sleep better? Is it to stop feeling sick all the time? Whatever your reasons are for trying the keto diet, or any other diet, make sure you know exactly what you want. You will have an easier time putting together and moving towards your goals.

Having a dietitian can be a wonderful support system. They only want to help you live your best and healthy life—remember that.

Okay, now that we've covered what Ketosis is, broken down some myths, and explained some stuff, now it's time to really get into Ketosis. Specifically, what makes Ketosis: ketones.

Chapter 2: Ketones

The making of ketones in your body is essential to any keto diet. The keto diet is all about encouraging the production of them in your body, before putting your body in a state of Ketosis. When you avoid carbs and sugar for about ten to 12 hours, your body automatically starts to make them.

Ketones are a molecule. They're water soluble, and a fuel source. They're derived from fat, and hold a lot of energy, almost like a small energy pack. Ketosis is when your body starts using them as an energy source. The adaptation takes time, especially as your body gets more and more used to it.

There are three types of ketones produced. Acetoacetate is created first, then beta-hydroxybutyric acid, which is created from acetoacetate, and acetone, which is a side product of acetoacetate.

Get Yourself into Ketosis

Yes, if you follow the guidelines for your diet set out in this book, you will find yourself eventually getting into Ketosis. Eating a low-carb diet will get you there—it's just a matter of time. However, there are times when you just want that push into it. Here are some things you can do to speed up the process:

1) *Coconut oil.* Coconut oil is all the rage these days. It is used on everything, from our hair to our skin. But there aren't that many people out there using coconut oil for what it was intended: cooking. Coconut oil contains fats called medium-chain triglycerides (MCT) which are absorbed very quickly and taken straight to the liver. They are immediately put to work, and converted into ketones and energy for you to burn. Implement coconut oil into your diet slowly. Go from one teaspoon per day to two to three tablespoons per day for about a week. You can use it for cooking, put it into recipes, you name it.

2) *More exercise.* Exercise is often about burning away these glycogen stores, and they'll always go first. They are your body's preferred source of energy, after all. The fewer glycogen stores, the faster you get into Ketosis. Pretty simple, right? Also, because it takes one to four weeks for your body to adjust to burning fats, physical performance might decrease for that period.

3) *Try a short fast or fat fast.* Quick note: your body has likely already been in a state of Ketosis. It often goes into Ketosis in between meals. When you burn away all your glucose/glycogen stores, your body feeds on its fat stores. Just consider putting yourself on a schedule of when you eat during the day. You could also consider a fat fast. A fat fast is where you go three to five days where you only eat 1,000 calories. 90% of these calories come from fat.

The quickest, easiest and most important healthiest way to enter Ketosis is to cut your carbs and up your fat intake. It will be difficult, and it may take some time, but it will be 100% worth it.

When you start producing ketones and getting into the state of Ketosis, there are a few ways of telling that you're there. Here's a list:

How To Know When You're In Ketosis

It can be a bit confusing as to whether or not you're even in Ketosis. If you're not sure, these signs are great ways to tell you if you're on track:

4) Bad breath. People often report bad breath following the ketone diet. It is caused by acetone and takes on a sweet, fruity smell. Ketogenic dieters brush their teeth more often and chew sugar-free gum. If you decide to chew gum, check for carbs on the nutrition label. For teeth brushers, consider getting a travel size and keep in your car or bag at all times.

5) Weight loss. At the beginning of a keto diet, you'll experience significant weight loss in a short amount of time. This is not fat being shed, but rather stored carbs and water. After the initial water drop, weight loss should occur consistently. This, of course, depends on you sticking to the diet and your calorie deficit.

6) Loss of appetite. Scientists are still unsure as to why this is, and more research is being done every day. One hypothesis is that it's due to increased protein and vegetable intake. On the keto diet, you're much more aware of what you're eating and are probably eating healthier than you did before. Because you're eating better, you're not as hungry anymore. It could also be the newly made ketones in your blood. They may be able to affect your brain and suppress your appetite.

7) Increased thirst. As the body starts repelling excess water, sodium, and carbs, you might find yourself peeing a lot. You also will find yourself very thirsty. Sip on water throughout the day to make yourself feel better.

8) Increased focus and more energy. Constantly being tired, feeling as if your brain is full of clouds, and feeling nauseous are all symptoms of the early stages of the keto diet. These

issues often lead people to give up. After they get through this initial state, though, ketogenic dieters report more energy and focus. Their mindset has become sharper. To get to this, your body must adapt to the changes in what it's getting for fuel. The ketones in your blood are helping your brain (which is 60% fat!) and making it work better. Ketones can also help with brain diseases and conditions, like concussions and memory loss. They can stabilize blood sugars, which could also help your brain.

9) Short-term tiredness. Being tired sucks. It especially sucks when it is your diet that is making you tired—when feeding your body should have the opposite effect. Tiredness is the biggest short-term issue for newly ketogenic dieters. It often causes people to give up. Who wants to be tired all the time? This is totally natural. Your body is adjusting to the fact that it's getting a new kind of fuel. It's like you're remaking your entire body's energy system, switching from one source to another. The majority of your body's energy is going to do that. This process can last anywhere from seven days to four weeks. To help yourself get through this, consider picking up some electrolyte supplements of sodium, magnesium, and potassium.

10) Short-term decrease in performance. Again, your body is used to running off one energy source. It has to adjust. This leads to tiredness, but also performance issues, at work and in exercise. The reduction of your glycogen stores, which up until now was your body's fuel source and the most efficient fuel source it has, leads to having to work harder to find these other fuel sources, such as your fat stores. It's like sore muscles; it needs to work at getting stronger, and as you do it more, it will get stronger. After several weeks, it will go to work again, and work better than it used to! You'll find yourself with more energy and the ability to do more than you used to.

11) Digestive system issues. The digestive system does not like change (at first). It gets used to what it's getting. It knows what to expect. By changing your diet, especially to something like the keto diet, you're majorly changing what it gets. This leads to issues like constipation and diarrhea. They might subside after a few weeks, but be mindful of what you're eating. Make sure you're getting a ton of low-carb, full of fiber veggies. Don't let yourself eat the same thing over and over again, even if you're doing the keto diet. A diverse palate will not only keep you from getting bored but will also decrease risks of digestive issues and nutrient deficiencies.

12) Insomnia, or Restless Sleep. This is another thing that tends to happen in the first few weeks. Many people who first start the keto diet report that they can't fall asleep, or they wake up several times over the course of a night. This should improve after a few weeks. There are no studies as to why this is, but it might be because your body is working extra hard to digest and use the fuel you're giving your body.

If you find yourself with these symptoms, you're very likely in some form of Ketosis. If you're still unsure, think of it this way: as long as you're following guidelines and your diet, you should be in Ketosis. If you're losing weight, enjoying yourself, and feeling healthy, no need to worry.

However, if you still want to know then consider a scientific test.

Tests

Measuring the ketones in your body with medical tests can be very useful. It will help you figure out when you feel best, and what is working for you and what is not. Using tests to monitor your Ketosis level is popular among people who are using the ketogenic diet.

There are three individual tests: blood, urine, and breath. All of them have pros and cons, and it's up to you to decide which one works for you.

Blood tests are the most accurate. They measure the ketone level in your blood and can tell you where you are in your ketone level. On the downsides, they can be very expensive and involve pricking your finger for blood. If you're a squeamish person, you might not want to. But if you think you could get used to it, try it out.

Urine tests are inexpensive and widely available. They're easy to use, almost like a pregnancy test, and non-invasive. Unfortunately, they are much less accurate. Urine is a waste product, meaning it's flushing out all of the stuff in your system. If you have ketones in your urine, this means that they're unused and unneeded. As your body uses more ketones for energy, you'll have less in your urine.

The last option is a breath test. Similar to a breath test for alcohol, it's a small, one-time purchase device, and it's very easy to use. It's the newest technology, so it does have limited research. Similar to urine, it's much less accurate than blood. It measures acetone, which relates to low blood ketone levels.

Ketone Supplements

One option is to help put your body in a Ketosis state is to try ketone supplements, which are called exogenous ketones. This means they're not made inside your body—rather they come from an external source. They're made in a lab and put in supplement form for you to try them. You find them in health stores.

Sometimes maintaining a steady ketogenic state just isn't realistic. Maybe it's your lifestyle, or maybe you slipped off the rails for a bit on vacation with your family. Either or, sometimes people just can't do it all the time. This is why people often take supplements; they can be a huge help in pushing you into that Ketosis state. You can do it right away—rather than wait a few days for your body to slip into it.

There are several different kinds of ketone supplements. Some of them taste all right, but they often don't taste very good. Be aware of the fact that often products will be listed as a ketone product, but actually don't do anything. Raspberry ketones are a very popular product on the market, but they actually don't work. Unfortunately, you'll find these products often.

It's not a bad idea to do your own research into ketone products. Don't fall for any advertising claims, and don't put anything into your body if you don't know exactly what's in it, and how it will help you reach that state of Ketosis.

So, that's it. That's pretty much all the scientific stuff about Ketosis, without too much scientific mumbo jumbo thrown in there. Now you should've grasped what Ketosis and ketones are. However, you may still be on the fence as to whether or not you want to embrace ketones into your lifestyle. Seeing as we are going to talk about the benefits of the keto diet, we're also going to talk about one of the biggest drug epidemics hitting North America right now: sugar.

Chapter 3: Benefits of Ketosis

The biggest reason why many people look towards the keto diet is weight loss. They want to lose weight and look good for the beach next summer. They also want to feel better about themselves, and embrace the idea of being able to go through their day without worrying about how they look and how people feel. With a lot of diets, this is the only benefit they have.

People choosing their diet based only on weight loss can lead to poor choices. When looking for a diet, people almost always just focus on this benefit. Losing weight is a great thing, especially if it's something you work hard for. Things such as exercise and eating healthy are some of the easiest ways to prevent conditions like kidney failure and heart disease. However, you should lose weight in a way that is good for you and your body. Your diet should have more than just that one benefit.

One reason this is a bad benefit—if weight loss is the sole reason for why you've picked a certain diet—is that it's not sustainable. At the end of the day, you're eventually going to reach your weight loss goal. What else will keep you going after this? What will drive you to completely embrace the lifestyle so that you keep the weight off permanently? Diets only work long term if you keep going at them, long after you've reached your weight goal and continue on the healthy lifestyle you're now in.

This is what makes the keto diet different. Once you completely immerse yourself in a state of Ketosis, you're now experiencing a host of other benefits besides weight loss. You become addicted to all of the other amazing benefits, not just the weight loss. Things like more energy to run around, skin without any blemishes, and just in general feeling so much better about yourself and your body, regardless of how much weight you've lost.

The weight loss is pretty great. Nobody's saying otherwise. The keto diet comes with quite a bit of weight loss. In the first week, people report up to ten pounds lost. This isn't fat losses, to be clear; this is the excess water and carbs in your body getting shed and being used up for energy. After this initial weight loss, you should be losing about one to two pounds a week, which is usually the amount that is considered healthy. This is great, but there is a host of other benefits to the keto diet. After all, there's a reason why celebrities like Kourtney Kardashian and LeBron James have sung the diet's praises.

One of the biggest reasons that diets often fail is because of appetite control. It can be hard to resist foods that you've always enjoyed, especially if you're already hungry. We've all been super hungry and eaten way more than we were supposed to. Well, good news— the keto diet helps with appetite control. It helps you make better choices in how much you need, or what you need. There are people on the keto diet who find themselves trying intermittent fasting, where you eat at select times and the rest of the time you don't. This is all thanks to the fact that they're better able to focus and say no.

Speaking of focus, people on the keto diet have an easier time doing just that, in work, at home, and otherwise. Their work production levels are higher—being able to get things done rather than procrastinating. When you're fueling your body with carbs, you don't realize just how much they're affecting your focus and making your brain feel foggy. The reason? Carbs cause blood sugars to rise and fall like crazy, and the energy source is not a consistent wave of energy. Ketones, on the other hand, are a consistent and steady battery that won't run out so easily.

Your energy levels go up because your body can only store so much glycogen (what glucose turns into when it's stored). You need to be storing and refueling yourself with more constantly. Your body can store much more fat; ergo, can store more energy in the form of fats rather than carbs. Is this why many athletes have turned to the diet to help them get through the day feeling like 100 bucks.

By eliminating many sugars from your diet, you're also reversing any issues with your pancreas and insulin production, meaning you're no longer at risk for Type 2 Diabetes. Type 2 Diabetes is one of these conditions that is very preventable and is caused by eating so much sugar that your pancreas goes into overdrive production trying to take care of it all. The keto diet is the opposite of this.

Another great health benefit of the keto diet is that it increases cholesterol. Yes, you may be panicking at reading that word as it's often associated with bad things, but we're not talking about that cholesterol. Your body produces two kinds: good and bad. Good cholesterol is called HDL, which carries cholesterol to the liver, where it can be reused and/or extracted. LDL is the bad cholesterol, which carries cholesterol to the rest of the body. The keto diet encourages the good cholesterol and reduces the amount of bad cholesterol. This reduces the chance of heart problems.

Another thing that helps reduce the chance of heart problems is having low blood pressure, which is another side effect of the keto diet. High blood pressure is often caused by too many carbs and sodium in your diet, and can be detrimental to your health. Having a steady, well-adjusted blood pressure is good for you.

The keto diet has also shown to have health benefits for some health conditions. These include epilepsy, Type 2 Diabetes, metabolic syndrome, and more. There are still many studies going on looking more into this, but it's not a bad idea to talk to your doctor if you have this or any other health issue. Do your own research into whether or not it may help.

The effect of the keto diet isn't just internal; it's external too. Keto dieters prone to acne might find themselves with clearer skin. Thanks to the fact that they're no longer eating large amounts of sugar, carbs, and glucose, all of which have been linked to bad skin, your skin could very well clear up. You'll be more confident and won't fear waking up with a giant pimple on your forehead.

The Bad Effect of Too Much Sugar

The keto diet is a very restrictive diet. Nobody is denying that. If you want to follow it properly, you have to cut out many foods that you probably very much enjoy, like candy bars, white bread, and even some (but not all) alcoholic beverages. You find yourself looking at nutritional labels a whole lot more, and having to put things back on the shelf because, well, it's got too many carbs. Carbs break down into glucose the same way in the bloodstream, so having too much of them will have the same effects on your body. It's not fun to do so— at least for the first little while.

However, to be fair, most of the foods that you'll end up cutting out, most of which have high amounts of sugar and carbs (which just turn into glucose) in them, are probably foods that you should be cutting out anyway. Glucose, which is often listed as another word for sugar, is actually found on many labels of candy at the supermarket, often in the first few ingredients (when listing ingredients, they're always put in the order of how much there is). However, sugar is not just found in candy; it is also found in tomato sauce, granola, and canned soup—it's literally everywhere.

Eating sugar is not just about weight gain and teeth decay, both of which are the main thing that people worry about eating too much of it. It's practically just another form of smoking, the new smoking, per se. It changes the structure of our cells the same way that smoking does, and strains the entire body when we eat it. It's not just about weight gain; it hurts every part of our body.

Your brain responds to sugar the same way it would cocaine. When you eat sugar, the chemical levels relating to happiness, dopamine, and serotonin rise in your brain. Just like cocaine, you want more after you come down from the high. How many times have you eaten a cookie, and an hour later immediately wanted another cookie?

Other immediate effects after having sugar are your insulin spikes, trying to deal with all the excess glucose in your blood. This leads to an eventual sugar crash, where you may find yourself feeling moody and drained and tired. In fact, eating a lot of sugar will often lead to you feeling very tired. Your body is constantly sending out insulin to help break it down. Add this to the fact that you are not getting the nutrients you need to energize your body means that you're going to be tired from eating so much sugar.

Long term, sugar can, of course, lead to obesity. But it's much worse than that. Sugar can change your cell structure, leading to them being able to resist the normal effects of insulin. It is not really understood why this happens. Your pancreas struggles to keep up with and absorb all the glucose in your bloodstream. Eventually, it becomes unable to keep up, and your blood sugar levels go higher and higher. There is excess glucose in your bloodstream, and it leads to Type 2 Diabetes.

Your liver also feels it. A healthy liver is essential to living a long and healthy life. Your body needs it, and it has many functions. One of these is that it regulates the blood sugar in your body, and helps fill up your energy reserves. When you need energy for later, it releases the stores back into the bloodstream. It can only store so much, however, and a surplus of it will turn into fat deposits. This can lead to liver disease. Fatty liver disease, where your liver holds more fat than it can metabolize, can develop within five years and can happen even quicker based on dietary habits.

Finally, your arteries. Blood that is weighed down and saturated with sugar can cause huge damage to all of them. They can't handle the amount and think of your arteries like plumbing, and sugar like a huge amount of sludge. Your pipes are going to get tired pumping all that sludge. It can lead to heart disease, kidney failure, strokes, and a huge number of issues for yourself down the road.

Even if you choose not to pursue the keto diet, seriously consider lessening how much sugar you're putting in your body. Seriously, it could save your life.

The unfortunate part is that sugar is virtually everywhere. There are many foods (like tomato sauce) that have sugar in them, and you might not even know it. To cut down on your sugar intake, start looking at nutritional labels and cut out things like candy bars and soda. That's a good start.

The Truth about the "Dangers" of Low-Carb Diets

Right alongside the "no carb" movement, there came a slew of well-meaning health professionals protesting it. Article upon articles were published on how carbs are good for you, followed by a wave of research to prove it. Carbs aren't the problem, scientists insisted; it's the fact that we need to eat good carbs.

This is true. We need good carbs in our diet, and even in the keto diet, you're still getting some. We need the glycogen to repair muscles and do things like work out. No one is saying that you need to cut carbs out completely. There is a difference between no carbs and low carbs.

Unfortunately, a whole lot of studies have been published, all about how dangerous low-carb diets are. Most people take them at face value, read the headline, and stuff their faces full of carbs, way overdoing it. They get scared off from trying the ketogenic diet entirely. Well, you're going to want to hear this: they're full of hooey.

Most health professionals who steer people away from the ketogenic diet mean well, but they probably don't know that much about it. Like we covered earlier, of course, some people should not be on a diet at all. The majority, though, would benefit in terms of their health.

Many articles railing against the keto diet will often list its side effects, but the majority of them are temporary and manageable. Once your body becomes accustomed to being reliant on a new fuel source, they become a distant memory, and you don't have to worry anymore.

As for these scientific studies that show that a low-carb diet isn't good for you, well, look a little closer. Most of these studies consider a "low-carb diet" to be 40% of their participants' daily calorie intake. That is not a low-carb diet. Many people who follow low-carb diets would agree that 40% of your calories coming from carbs is a moderate-to-high intake. Researchers should really be basing their research on actual low-carb diets.

Usually, when scientists do choose to have a study based on an actual ketogenic diet, what do they use? Rats. They use rats. Rodents are not people, and it is baffling to see just how easily people are willing to swallow studies done on other creatures other than ourselves. People should not be eating based on the effects that ketogenic rat food has on mice, rats, and other rodents.

If you're really nervous about trying a ketogenic diet, after listing all the benefits, do your own research. Don't just look at the headlines. This is a problem in our society where we constantly take all our information from just that one sentence. Headlines can often be very misleading (this is mostly due to websites wanting to get more clicks, not a genuine desire to mislead people). If you want to look more into the studies of the risks of low-carb diets, read the studies and know what they did to get these results. You may learn something.

So we've covered pretty much all you need to know about the diet. We've covered the science, myths, benefits, and how low-carb diets are good for you. Now it's time to get started preparing for your journey. The first step to this? Figuring out your macro count.

Chapter 4: Macros

Calorie counting is considered a staple in nearly every single diet. Its baseline is pretty simple: you count the number of calories you eat, so you know where to stop or where to get to. By keeping track of your calories, you're knowing how much you're eating, and how much you need to eat to keep within your goals.

The keto diet is slightly different in that regard. With many diets, you really just need to focus on the calories. You don't have to worry too much about anything else if your only goal is to lose weight. In the keto diet, you also have to count macros as well. What are macros?

We already went over them a bit in Chapter 1, but macros are the three main nutrients that should make up every meal: carbohydrates, fats, and protein. In every healthy diet, you should be getting a certain amount of each of these. It's like how your mom told you growing up that you needed to fill half your plate with green veggies. That's actually pretty true.

The difference between the keto diet and just any old diet is that you really need to focus on these macros. Calories are important too, but macros are especially important. Now we're going to talk about them, and we're going to go over what their specific role is in our diet, and why they're important.

Carbs

Carbs are considered the bad guy in the keto diet, and ketogenic dieters put a lot of time and effort into avoiding them. But we can't avoid them completely, which is a big mistake that many beginner keto dieters make. We need carbs, whether we like it or not. We don't need nearly as many as we eat, but we still need them. Important bodily functions like our liver and our kidneys use glucose to fuel them so they can do their jobs, and even our brains need a little shot of glucose.

Another reason we can't quit carbs? Fiber. Fiber is essential to any healthy diet, and it goes hand in hand with carbs. Look at the nutritional label, and you'll see fiber right underneath carbohydrates. Fiber is incredibly important for our digestive health, helping us feel full and improves good cholesterol. For men, you need an average of about 30 grams a day, and for women 24 grams. Fiber also doesn't get counted the same as macros. This is because fiber isn't digested the same way most nutrients are. Instead, it's used and discarded. The fiber count in your diet won't count towards your overall carbs.

Picking what carbs will make up that 5% can be tricky, but soon it will be second nature. It's about being able to read nutrition labels and look at ingredient lists. Look for ingredients such as glucose, galactose, fructose, sucrose, lactose, and maltose. These are all forms of simple sugars often found on ingredient boxes, and the ones you should be avoiding. You want complex sugars, like starch, in your diet. Starch is found in many fruits and vegetables, and many of them are perfect for the keto diet.

There is a whole section next chapter about foods you can eat on the keto diet, but for now, think of leafy greens, legumes, and fruits. These are healthy examples of fiber, and good choices of carbs to eat. However, think of anything that is high in fiber, high in nutrients, and low calorie. If you stick to these rules, you should be fine.

Protein

If you're brand spanking new to the ketogenic diet, protein will be the one thing that won't have too much of a difference. Your intake will stay pretty much the same.

Protein is important because of how much it does for your body. It basically helps build a massive proportion of it, such as your hair and your nails, and behaves as the foundation for things like blood, bones, muscles, skin, and bone cartilage. Protein is also essential in the production of enzymes, hormones, and other body chemicals.

Protein is also needed for your body rebuilding itself when it's injured. It repairs sore muscles, reducing muscle loss, helping build lean muscle, and curb hunger. When you eat, it is thanks to protein that you will be feeling full.

Your body does not store protein the same way it does carbs and fats, which is why you need to keep up with eating it. After a hard workout, it will be the protein that will get your recovery moving faster. Picking healthy, plant-based or, otherwise, protein sources will help you feel good and like you can conquer the world.

Fats

With any keto diet, fats are where it's at. Out of all the macros, fats are the most calorically dense of all of them. There are about nine calories per gram of fat, while both other macros have an average of about four calories. This will, of course, depend on the food you are sourcing it from.

Fat is a reserve for energy storage in the body. In the days of cave dwellers, when there could be weeks between meals, it was used as an energy store to keep our ancestors going through the weeks. Believe it or not, several thousand years ago, it was considered attractive to be overweight and have a lot of fat stored away for these hard times. Fat is what provides us with a layer of insulation for our organs and keeping our body temperature up. Fat also plays an important role in our cellular and hormonal health and is one of the primary sources of energy for our brains. It keeps our skin soft and healthy.

Like we said before, fat does get a bad rap in the dieting world. The lie of the "zero fat" or "no fat" product has only strengthened it. Just stick to the healthy fats, and you'll be burning these ketones in no time.

Measuring Your Calories and Macros

Now that we know and understand macros, and the importance of protein, carbs, and fat, now it's time to measure how much of them we need. The basic guidelines of the keto diet, 75% fat, 20% protein, and 5% carbs are usually a rough estimate. It will depend on person to person, and even the calculations done here are only a ballpark rate.

It will be up to you to pay attention to your body, to figure out what's working and what isn't, depending on your goals. If you want to lose weight and it's not happening, you can adjust your calorie rate. If you're hoping to build up some muscle and lifting weights isn't getting any easier, you're going to have to up your protein intake. Paying attention to your body is essential to any healthy lifestyle.

Before you begin the keto diet, you need to calculate the following:

1) Basal Metabolic rate (BMR)

2) Your total energy expenditure

3) Know your body fat percentages and lean mass

4) Adjust your calorie intake for weight loss or weight gain (or skip this step entirely if this isn't one of your goals)

5) Calculate your carb intake

6) Calculate your protein intake

7) Calculate your fat intake

This may sound like a lot of math. You probably were not expecting that. However, this math is only a small part of your journey, and all of it can be done with a calculator. If you don't have one with you right now, there are apps for that. There are also many places online that will calculate the rate for you, but you might just want to do it yourself. All of the basic math equations are done below. The only numbers you'll really need are your body weight, your height, and your age.

Easy peasy.

Your Basal Metabolic Rate

The Basal Metabolic Rate, or BMR as we'll be referring to it from now on, is the number of calories your body needs to do what it needs to do. Things like breathing, sleeping, eating food—all the basic things that you do every day without thinking. Everything you do burns calories and the BMR is the magic number we need to do these things without it being a strain on the body. The more mass you have, the more calories you need.

You can't get an exact rate. You'll never get to know the precise number that you need. All you'll be able to get is a rough rate, and as long as you stick in the ballpark of this number, you should be fine. The closest formula that comes close is the Harris-Benedict equation. It's considered the best way to figure out your metabolic rate and is the equation many dieticians, doctors, and nutritionists use.

For Men: $66 + (6.2 \times \text{current weight in pounds}) + (12.7 \times \text{height in inches}) - (6.76 \times \text{age}) = \text{BMR}$

For Women: $65.1 + (4.35 \times \text{current weight in pounds}) + (4.7 \times \text{height in inches}) - (4.7 \times \text{age}) = \text{BMR}$

If you're on the metric system, you better go for the Mifflin-St. Jeor Formula. It will be much easier for you.

For Men: 10 × weight in kilograms + 6.25 × height in centimeters - 5 × age in years + 5 = BMR

For Women: 10 × weight in kilograms + 6.25 × height in centimeters - 5 × age in years + 161 = BMR

Again, all of these equations can be done on a calculator. The numbers will come from your age, weight, and height, and also be influenced by your gender. Why?

For your gender, men's and women's bodies have different compositions and different builds.

Age because muscle mass declines after you hit 30, and that means your BMR decreases as well.

Your height and body weight because the bigger you are, the more energy you need.

Your Total Daily Energy Expenditure

Your total daily energy expenditure (TDEE) is based on the amount of energy you're doing. At this point, it's a good idea to be realistic. Planning to exercise and actually exercising are two different things. We're going to talk more about exercise later, but for now, just base it on how much exercise you're currently doing—no shame if you're not doing any! That can always be changed later. None of these numbers are permanent. Just be honest with yourself. These numbers will not work if you lie.

Multiply these numbers by your BMR, depending on which category you fit into.

1.2 = little to no exercise

1.375 = light exercise, one-three days a week

1.55 = moderate exercise, three-five days a week

1.725 = hard exercise, six-seven days a week

1.9 = very intense exercise, seven days a week

If you have a career that is physically demanding, like construction or one that involves walking a lot like retail or restaurant work, take this into consideration.

Your Body Fat Percentage

Measuring your body fat percentage is how you know the amount of body fat you have. Anything left over is your lean body mass. It will help decipher how much protein you need to maintain or build your muscle mass. Muscle burns more calories than fat even when it's doing absolutely nothing.

Your fat percentages can be measured in several different ways. It will all depend on you, your budget, and what you're comfortable with.

DEXA Scan: this is the closest you'll get to an accurate body fat percentage. It's an X-ray experience that measures your bone mineral density. While it is the most accurate way, it is expensive and can be very time-consuming.

Skinfold Calipers: These are the easiest to get a hold of and the most recommended. They're easily available at any doctors and gyms. Just head up to the counter the next time you're there and ask. If for some reason they do not have them or don't offer the service, they are not too expensive online and are available at many different retailers. They're also an investment, so if you're someone who plans on measuring your body fat a lot, these are definitely something to look into.

Body measurements: This is not the most accurate reading, but it is generally easy and can be done at home. All you need is a measuring tape, and to measure the neck, waist, height, etc. It will give you a good estimate. Here's what you should do:

Height: make sure you're barefoot and standing up straight.

Neck: look ahead, relax your shoulders, but no hunching. If you're a man, the tape should be placed below your Adam's apple.

Waist: the tape needs to be placed around the waist, the narrowest part of the abdomen for women and at the belly button for men. The best result you'll get is if someone else does it for you and your arms hang at your side. Breathe in and exhale slowly, and measure after you release the breath.

Hips: they should be measured at the widest part of the hip or butt.

You're going to get your most accurate measurements if someone else does it for you. It should also be done in the morning before breakfast. If you want to get a very accurate number, you could do it a few days in a row and choose the average.

Once you have gotten these measurements, head on over to the internet and look for a "body fat calculator". It's also called the Navy Body Fat Calculator. There are many different ones to try. Type in these numbers, and they'll give you your body fat percentage.

Eye it: Again, this is not going to be the exact, accurate number. Body fat percentages can be eyed—you just need a mirror and a bathing suit.

Look at our guide.

Stand in front of a mirror with your shirt off. Eye your abdomen, turn around and look at your butt, then your face. Consult the list below to find which one matches you best.

Men

Men have a lower body percentage than woman do, and carry most of their fat around their abdomen.

5% to 9%: this is not sustainable or considered healthy for most men. At this percentage, every single muscle is showing, with very little to no confusion, and veins are visible and clear. You'll often find this body in bodybuilders at the peak of the competition season.

10% to 14%: this is the body that people think of when they think "beach body" and is the body most men will strive for. There is a clear separation between muscles, but not all of them. Veins will show mostly in the arms and the legs.

15% to 19%: this look is very lean. There is little definition of the muscles and almost no clear separation between them. It is nearly nonexistent.

20% to 24%: this is the average body that the majority of men have. The separation between the muscles is not at all there, and there is a bit of fat around the stomach. However, it is not rounded.

25% to 29%: anywhere above this is considered obese. The waist is bigger, and the stomach starts rounding out. There may be a little neck fat.

30% to 34%: the fat has distributed more around the body. The waist is large around the hips.

35% to 39%: the stomach will have a clear protrusion and hang. It will grow over 40 inches.

Women

Women, as a rule, have a higher body fat percentage than men do. They carry more fat in their breasts, thighs, and butt.

10% to 14%: usually found in bodybuilders at the peak of competition and is not sustainable or healthy for long periods. The less vascularity, the father from 10%.

15 % to 19%: this percentage is usually found in fitness and bikini models. There is less shape to the hips, thighs, and butts because of the lack of body fat. There is little clear definition of muscles in the arms and legs, along with some visible veins.

20% to 24%: There is less separation of the muscles, and the majority of female athletes fall into this range. You're considered highly fit, and this is usually the body that women wish they had.

There will be less definition in the arms and legs, with most of it in the abdominal muscles.

25% to 29%: the average woman falls into this range. Curves form around hips, and there is more fat in the thighs and the butt.

30% to 34%: there is more fat in the hips, butt, and thighs. They will be more rounded and pronounced.

35% to 39%: the face and the neck starts to gain fat, and the waist will be over 32 inches. The belly will often start rounding out.

40% to 44%: the thighs and the hips become very large, and the waist will be typically 35 inches.

45% to 50%: the waist will be over 35 inches, and the hips will be wider than the shoulders. The skin often loses its smoothness and will likely dimple.

When you've finally determined your body fat percentage, you can use this to figure out your lean body mass.

Body weight in pounds × point percentage (ex; if your body fat percentage is 25 then it will be .25) = pounds of body fat.

To figure out your body lean mass, take the pounds of body fat and subtract it from your original body weight. That is your lean body mass, and you can use it to figure out how much protein you need. You can also use the above information to decide what your goal is, and where you want to be in your fat loss journey.

Adjusting Your Calorie Intake

If you're not looking to lose weight, skip this step.

The idea is to eat fewer calories than you are eating to maintain your current, at this very moment, weight. For just starting off, take off only about 10% to 20% of your intake. If you wish, you may take off more, but you might find that it's harder to keep within that range. It's also not recommended to take off more than 30% for a long period.

To get this number, do this equation below:

(TDEE × point whatever percentage, if you're talking of 10%, it will be .10) - original calorie count = amount of calories to eat every day.

If you wish to gain muscle, you will need a few more calories. A 5% to 10% increase will help but remember: it will only work if you work out as well.

(Calorie expenditure × .05) + calorie expenditure = calorie surplus

Calorie counting can be tough, especially if you're not used to it. There are several apps out there that are designed to help people do this, and there will be some tips later on regarding how to make it as easy as it can be. However, good news—counting macros is considered more important than counting calories in the keto diet.

Carb Intake

You already know now that the keto diet is a low-carb one. You've already been told that 5% is generally the average amount of calories you will be getting from carbs, but it's really up to you to decide. If you want to put yourself into Ketosis as soon as possible, go for the 5%. If you want to work your way down, gradually cutting out carbs until you hit that 5%, do that. Some people choose to have 10% be their number. It's really up to you.

Most people need about 20 to 50 grams per day. Remember: your total net carbs will equal your total carb count minus the amount of fiber you consume. To calculate this:

TDEE × the percentage of calories you've decided ÷ 4 = the number of carbs in grams you should be eating per day

As long as you keep your carb levels in the 5% to 10% range, you should be able to get into Ketosis no problem. However, if you find yourself struggling to enter the sweet spot where you start to burn fat, consider lowering your carb intake.

Keep this in mind: when counting carbs, there is a difference between counting carbs and counting net carbs. Net carbs are basically the grams of total carbs in a food, minus the fiber. Fiber does not get absorbed by the body in the same way that other nutrients do, meaning that it doesn't raise your blood sugar levels or trigger insulin. So, when you do count your carbs for the day, make sure to subtract the carbs caused by fiber.

Protein

Protein should make up about 20% to 25% of your calories in the average, standard ketogenic diet. If you're having a difficult time entering Ketosis, too much protein may very well be the problem. This is a common mistake for beginners.

If you're not someone who is active, .6 to .8 grams of protein per pound of lean mass every day will do it.

If you fall into the moderately - lightly active category, .8 to 1 gram protein per lean body mass pound every day is for you.

If you are working towards gaining muscle, increase that number to 1 to 1.2 grams per pound of lean body mass.

Once you've figured out how much protein you need, use this formula:

range × 4 = number of calories you need

For example, if you have a lean body mass of 130 pounds and you're not active, you'll need between 90 and 104 grams of protein per day. Multiply 90 by 4, and you get 360, which would be the number of calories you need.

Fats

Finally, we come to fats. Fats will make up whatever percentage is left over from the other two, but it's usually about 70% to 80% of your daily calorie count. Add the protein and carb percentage you've decided together, and subtract it from 100. That is what your fat needs.

People are often surprised at how much fat they need to consume in the keto diet but just remember: it will all be worth it in the end. The benefits will come pouring in, and you'll feel and look great.

There is no guarantee they will be 100% accurate, so don't worry too much about that. Don't let yourself go there. The goal here is to have a range number to work with. The first few steps to any new lifestyle or diet are to figure out what works for you along the way until you are fully accustomed to the idea.

Chapter 5: Nutrition

Nutrition is a big deal in the keto diet. It's not just about eating a lot of fat; it's about measuring just how much you're eating. Keeping track is very important, especially if you want to get into Ketosis as quickly as possible. Here is a list, along with their nutrition information, but keep in mind that you'll probably want to look at the foods' actual nutrition labels. This will give you an idea, but of course, the number will vary depending on the brand.

Meats

Meats are a staple food in keto, and you'll have them in many of your meals. Meats have no to very little carbs and contain many vitamins and nutrients you need, such as vitamin B, potassium, selenium, and zinc. It is also a valuable source of high-quality protein.

To get the most of the benefits of your cuts, stick to free-range and grass-fed. They contain more omega-3 fats and more antioxidants.

	Portion	Calories	Fat	Carbs	Protein
Chicken	3 oz. (85 g)	187	11 g	0 g	20 g

Pork	3 oz. (85 g)	202	12 g	0 g	22 g
Steak	3 oz. (85 g)	236	16 g	0 g	22 g
Ground Beef	3 oz. (85 g)	231	15 g	0 g	23 g
Lamb	3 oz. (85 g)	250	18 g	0 g	21 g
Bacon	3 slices	161	12 g	0.6 g	12 g
Ham	3 oz. (85 g)	118	5 g	1 g	19 g
Turkey	3 oz. (85 g)	161	6.3 g	0.1 g	24 g
Sausage	2 links	150	13 g	0.7 g	8.5 g
Meatballs	4 (medium)	324	25 g	9.1 g	16 g
Roast Beef	20 g	23	0.7 g	0 g	3.7 g

Fats and Oils

Many of the oils listed here are pure fat sources and will help decrease heart disease risks. They're high in antioxidants and are a great addition to drizzle over low-fat foods for a bit of an extra fat boost.

	Portion Size	Calories	Fats	Carbs	Protein

Butter	1 Tbsp.	102	12 g	0 g	0.1 g
Coconut Oil	1 Tbsp.	121	13 g	0 g	0 g
Olive Oil	1 Tbsp.	119	14 g	0 g	0 g
Ghee	1 Tbsp.	112	13 g	0 g	0 g
Lard	1 Tbsp.	115	13 g	0 g	0 g
Avocado Oil	1 Tbsp.	124	14 g	0 g	0 g

Vegetables

While there are admittedly many vegetables that don't make the keto cut, there are many that do. All of these veggies are low in calories and carbs, as well as high in dietary fiber. It's important to get a lot of fiber, as it helps your digestive system and makes you feel full. Veggies also have a huge amount of nutrients and prevent heart disease and many different cancers.

	Portion Size	Calories	Fat	Carbs	Protein
Cauliflower	1 Cup (1" pieces)	29	1 g	5 g	2 g
Cabbage	1 Cup (shredded)	35	0 g	8 g	2 g
Avocado	1 fruit	227	21 g	12 g	2.7 g

Broccoli	1 Cup (chopped)	55	1 g	11 g	4 g
Zucchini	1 Cup (sliced)	27	1 g	5 g	2 g
Peppers	1 Cup (chopped/sliced)	38	0 g	9 g	1 g
Eggplants	1 Cup (1" cubed)	35	0.2 g	8.6 g	1 g
Tomatoes	1 Cup (chopped/slice)	32	0.4	7 g	1.6 g
Asparagus	5 spears	17	0.2 g	3.1 g	1.8 g
Cucumber	1 Cup (slices)	16	0.1 g	3.8 g	0.7 g
Mushroom	1 Cup (slices)	44	0.7	8.3 g	3.4 g
Onion	1 (medium)	41	0 g	9.5 g	1.3 g
Spinach	1 Cup	41	0.5 g	6.8 g	5.3 g
Lettuce	2 Cups (shredded)	16	0 g	7.5 g	1.2 g
Green Beans	10 beans	22	0 g	5 g	1.2 g
Olives	10 olives	44	4 g	2.4 g	0 g

Celery	2 stalks	20	0 g	4.5 g	0.9 g

Dairy

Dairy is not only nutritious and delicious, but it also fits right into the keto diet. Lots of cheeses are low in carbs but high in fat, and they contain conjugated linoleic acid fat, which is linked to fat loss and improvements in body composition. Plain Greek yogurt and cottage cheese are high in protein and promote feelings of fullness.

	Serving Size	Calories	Fat	Carbs	Protein
Heavy Cream	1 Tbsp. (fluid)	51	5.4 g	0.4 g	0.4 g
Regular Cream Cheese	2 Tbsp.	102	10 g	1.6 g	2 g
Sour Cream	1 Tbsp.	24	2.3 g	0.6 g	0 g
Blue Cheese	1 cubic inch	60	5 g	0 g	3.6 g
Gouda	1 oz.	101	8 g	0.6 g	7.1 g
Parmesan	1 Tbsp.	21	1.4 g	0.7 g	1.4 g
Swiss Cheese	1 cubic inch	59	4.6 g	0 g	4 g

Mozzarella	1 slice (1 oz.)	85	6.3 g	0.6 g	6.3 g
Brie	1 oz.	95	7.8 g	0 g	5.9 g
Muenster	1 slice (1 oz.)	103	8.4 g	0 g	6.6 g
Monterey Jack	1 slice (1 oz.)	104	8.5 g	0 g	6.9 g
Cottage Cheese	1 cup	213	9.4 g	7.4 g	24 g
Colby	1 slice (1 oz.)	110	9 g	0.7 g	6.7 g
Provolone	1 slice (1 oz.)	98	7.5 g	0.6 g	7.2 g
Greek Yogurt (Plain)	1 Cup	134	1 g	8.2	23 g

Nuts and Seeds

Nuts and seeds are full of healthy fats and have low carbs, as well as being high in fiber. Eating them has a ton of benefits, like reduced risks of cancers and heart disease. They're a great snack to have on hand when these cravings hit you.

	Portion Size	Calories	Fat	Carbs	Protein
Almonds (raw)	10 nuts	77	6.8 g	2.7 g	2.7 g
Peanuts (raw)	10 nuts	59	5 g	2.1 g	2.4 g
Almond Butter	1 Tbsp.	98	8.9 g	3 g	3.4 g
Peanut Butter	1 Tbsp.	94	7.9 g	3.8 g	3.5 g
Macadamia Nuts	5 nuts	93	9.8 g	1.8 g	1 g
Pecans	10 nuts	103	11 g	2.1 g	1.4 g
Hazelnuts	10 nuts	88	8.5 g	2.3 g	2.1 g
Walnuts	5 nuts	133	13 g	2.8 g	3.1 g
Sunflower Seeds	1 Tbsp.	44	4 g	1.2 g	1.5 g

Seafood

Fish are great for the keto diet because they're full of fats and rich in vitamins and minerals, like potassium. The majority of seafood is carb free, with a few exceptions like clams and other shellfish, but they can still be enjoyed in moderation.

Fish is also high in omega-3 fats. Omega-3 fats help maintain lower insulin levels and increase insulin sensitivity, meaning it's better able to do its job. It also has been linked to lower risks of many diseases and improved mental health.

	Portion Size	Calories	Fat	Carbs	Protein
Salmon	3 oz. (85 g)	175	10 g	0 g	19 g
Snapper	3 oz. (85 g)	109	1.5 g	0 g	22 g
Trout	3 oz. (85 g)	162	7.2 g	0 g	23 g
Tuna (fresh)	3 oz. (85 g)	111	0.5 g	0 g	25 g
Cod	3 oz. (85 g)	89	0.7 g	0 g	19 g
Catfish	3 oz. (85 g)	122	6.1 g	0 g	16 g
Halibut	3 oz. (85 g)	94	1.4 g	0 g	19 g
Clams	5 (small)	70	0.9 g	2.4 g	12 g
Oysters	3 (medium)	122	3.5 g	7.4 g	14 g
Lobster	1	233	3.2 g	5.1 g	43 g
Crab	3 oz. (85 g)	71	0.6 g	0 g	15 g
Scallops	5	72	0.6 g	3.5 g	13 g
Mussels	3 oz. (85 g)	146	3.8 g	6.3 g	20 g

Berries

Berries are a great way to get some sweetness in your life, especially since most fruits are just too high in carbs to eat on the keto diet.

They're full of antioxidants and tons of other good stuff. If you're someone with a sweet tooth, berries will be able to hit that spot that wants a candy bar.

	Portion Size	Calories	Fat	Carbs	Protein
Blueberries	1 Cup	84	0.5 g	21 g	1.1 g
Blueberries (Frozen)	1 Cup	79	1 g	19 g	0.7 g
Raspberry	1 Cup	64	0.8 g	15 g	1.5 g
Raspberry (Frozen)	1 Cup	73	0.9 g	17 g	1.7 g
Blackberries	1 Cup	62	0.7 g	14 g	2 g
Blackberries (Frozen)	1 Cup	90	0 g	22 g	2 g

Eggs

Eggs are not just a great option to include in a ketogenic breakfast, but also very healthy. When you eat eggs, make sure you eat the entire thing, including the yolk. The yolk has the most nutrients.

	Portion Size	Calories	Fat	Carbs	Protein
Egg (large)	1	72	4.8 g	0 g	6.3 g
Egg (medium)	1	63	4.2	0 g	5.5 g
Egg (small)	1	54	3.6 g	0 g	4.8

Sauces

Keep in mind that buying these store-bought sauces can be hit or miss. Some stores have "keto-friendly" options, which is not a bad thing to look for, but they're still pretty rare. It will really just be brand to brand. Just be sure to check these nutrient labels, and consider making some sauces at home.

	Serving Size	Calories	Fat	Carb	Protein
Caesar Dressing	1 Tbsp.	80	8.5 g	0.5 g	0 g
Ranch Dressing	1 Tbsp.	65	6.7 g	0.9 g	0 g
Alfredo Sauce	¼ Cup	269	25 g	3.9 g	7.1 g
Hot Sauce	1 Tsp.	1	0 g	0 g	0 g
Mayonnaise	1 Tbsp.	94	10 g	0 g	0 g

Drinks

Most issues with drinks, like coffee or tea, is all the stuff we add to them, such as sugar, sugary coffee creamers or any other kind of sweetener. And let's not forget there is always water.

	Serving Size	Calories	Fat	Carbs	Protein
Coffee	1 Cup (8 fl. oz.)	2	0 g	0 g	0 g
Tea	1 Cup (8 fl. oz.)	2	0 g	1 g	0 g

Seven-Day Meal Plan

Keep in mind that this does not have to be your "ride or die" strict meal plan. This is just a good example of what your first week on a diet will look like, and many weeks after. For the first week, you should be keeping your meals simple, built around the foods you love, without doing anything too crazy in the kitchen—especially if you're not well versed in cooking and only know the bare essentials. Think of this list as a guideline, not a hardcore "you must do it this way" meal plan.

Day 1

Breakfast: Eggs, scrambled, in butter or olive oil, on a bed of spinach or lettuce, topped with avocado

Snack: Nuts of your choice

Lunch: Spinach salad with salmon or chicken

Snack: Celery and pepper sticks, with guacamole for dipping

Dinner: Pork chop with mashed cauliflower and cabbage slaw

Day 2

Breakfast: Bulletproof coffee (coffee made with butter and oil, find the recipe below), with hard-boiled eggs

Snack: Nuts of your choice

Lunch: Tuna salad with tomatoes

Snack: Roast beef and sliced cheese roll-ups

Dinner: Zucchini or veggie noodles with meatballs, topped with cream sauce

Day 3

Breakfast: Cheese and veggie omelet with salsa on the side

Snack: Greek yogurt topped with crushed nuts of your choice

Lunch: Spinach salad with salmon or chicken

Snack: Smoothie made with almond milk, greens, almond butter, and protein powder

Dinner: Roasted chicken with sautéed greens and mushrooms

Day 4

Breakfast: Smoothie made with almond milk, greens of your choice, and nut butter of your choice, with berries

Snack: Two hard-boiled eggs

Lunch: Chicken on a bed of greens with your choice of cheese and veggies

Snack: Bell pepper slices with a side of sliced cheese

Dinner: Grilled shrimp topped with a butter sauce with a side of greens

Day 5

Breakfast: Fried eggs with bacon and a side of greens

Snack: Nuts of your choice with some berries of your choice

Lunch: Beef burger on a portobello mushroom or lettuce "bun" topped with avocado and a side of greens or salad

Snack: Celery sticks dipped in nut butter of your choice

Dinner: Baked chicken with broccoli and peppers, a side of cauliflower rice and with a sauce of your choice

Day 6

Breakfast: Baked eggs in avocado cups

Snack: Kale chips

Lunch: Tuna salad and tomatoes

Snack: Nuts of your choice

Dinner: Grilled steak with peppers and broccolini

Day 7

Breakfast: Eggs scrambled with veggies, topped with salsa

Snack: Dried seaweed strips and cheese

Lunch: Grilled chicken sandwich with a lettuce "bun" with a side of greens of your choice, topped with butter

Snack: Turkey jerky

Dinner: Broiled trout with butter and sautéed greens of your choice

Bulletproof Coffee

Bulletproof coffee is a great way to get a little extra fat in you to kick off your morning. You might have heard of it by its other names, such as keto coffee, fatty coffee, butter coffee, etc., but the gist of it is basically the same; it is coffee mixed with butter and oil. The extra fat helps satiety and curbs your cravings and will keep you from reaching for a huge breakfast. The mix of caffeine and the butter will give you an extra boost and help you more than just the caffeine would (you can use decaf if you wish).

The main oil in bulletproof coffee is usually MCT oil. MCT oil is the fastest absorbed oil and goes straight to the liver to be converted into ketones. MCT oil can be found online, but coconut oil is also a great substitution. If you don't have either of these, something like lard or ghee will also work. The best combination is about one part MCT oil/substitution to two parts butter.

If you're used to having sugar in your coffee, you can put other sweeteners in it, like cinnamon or a little bit of cocoa powder. A little bit of cinnamon is always a great addition to your coffee, but cocoa powder is better for you if you're only a diehard chocolate fan. It tends to be pretty bitter.

Directions:

1 Tbsp. MCT/Substitution

2 Tbsp. Butter

12 oz. coffee

Prepare coffee as you normally would. Pour the coffee, along with your other ingredients, in a blender. Blend on high for 30 seconds. Enjoy.

Calories: 320 Fat: 36 g Carbs: 0 g Protein: 0 g

Foods That Are Off Limits

- *Fruit*: apples, oranges, bananas, peaches, melons, pears, cherries, pineapples, grapefruit, plums, watermelon, etc.
- *Grains and Starches*: rice, oats, corn, barley, bulgur, buckwheat, quinoa, wheat, rye, corn, etc.

- *Grain Products*: cereal, bread, corn, oatmeal, flour, granola, popcorn, crackers, pizza, pasta
- *Low-Fat Dairy*: skim milk, skim cheese, fat-free yogurt, cream cheese
- *Root Vegetables*: carrots, yams, parsnips, turnips, beets, potatoes, sweet potatoes
- *Legume*s: kidney beans, black beans, navy beans, pinto beans, peas, chickpeas, soybeans, lentils
- *Sweeteners*: sugar, maple syrup, honey, agave syrup, Splenda, saccharin, Aspartame, corn syrup
- *Sweets*: candy, cookies, chocolate, cake, pies, tarts, pastries, pudding, custard, ice cream
- *Some Oils*: canola oil, peanut oil, soybean oil, grape seed oil, sesame oil, sunflower oil
- *Sweetened Drinks*: Juice, smoothies, soda, sweetened teas, and coffees
- *Sweetened Sauces and Dips*: ketchup, BBQ sauce, most tomato sauces, some salad dressings, and hot sauces

Keep in mind that many of the foods on this list are referring to their store-bought, prepackaged versions, especially with things like sauces. Tomato sauces from the store often have a ton of sugar in them, but ones made at home will depend on the recipe. Consider looking into making some things at home if you're not willing to give them up.

It may seem like this list is super long. And very restrictive. You might see several of your favorites and think "I definitely can't do this."

You can. You can do this. You absolutely, 100% can do this.

Instead of thinking of all the things you can't eat anymore, or at least must eat in very small quantities and very rarely, think of all the foods you can eat. There is an entire world of food and recipes out there, all of them delicious in their own way and all of them different. Cooking should be an adventure and something you enjoy.

Too often we see nutrition as something that is a chore. Taking care of your body, fueling your body with the energy it needs to really get to where it needs to be, that should be one of your greatest joys.

When you focus on your meals, really try to pick out foods that you love rather than foods you think you should have. Yes, giving your body nutrients is important, but you should be looking forward to your meals. Nobody wants to cook something and then not want to eat it. That sounds terrible.

Look at the list above. If there is something not on that list that you enjoy eating in some shape or form, well, that sounds a little crazy. Pick out the three ingredients from the list above, balancing the macros, and build a meal around them. Even throwing them all in a pan and swishing them around in some olive oil or butter counts.

If you're a beginner cook, stick to the three to five ingredient margins. Just focus on getting these macros right and learning about this journey. It won't be easy, but you'll get it done.

Easy Substitutions for Foods

When first switching over, it can definitely be a difficult road of trying to figure out how and what you can eat, and disappointing when you realize you're going to have to really cut out many foods you have probably enjoyed and are a large part of your diet, such as pasta, chips, and rice.

Thankfully, though, there are some substitutes out there that you can easily make staples of your diet, and, in many instances, taste better than their carb and sugar loaded alternatives, with more flavor and variety, on top of all their nutritional value.

Lettuce Leaves for Tortillas

Tortillas and tacos are awesome, but their shells are basically all carbs. Replace them with large lettuce leaves. The crunch is similar, and there is a massive cut in the calories you're consuming.

Cauliflower Rice for Rice

Rice is often at the center of several meals and is considered a staple in many households. It can be difficult to give it up. Cauliflower rice is a great alternative because it basically tastes the same, but the only issue is that the texture is much harder than regular rice. If you are picky about the texture of food, this may not be for you. All you have to do is grind it a bit in the food processor, but only for a few seconds as you don't want it to become all mashed up.

Almond Milk for Milk

Almond milk is not quite the same as regular milk. It doesn't have much creaminess, and you can especially notice that when you drink it plain. However, if you're drinking it in tea, mixing it into recipes, or eating it with cereal, you will hardly notice. There are generally two kinds of almond milk: sweetened and unsweetened. Always go for the unsweetened version. Almond milk can be made easily at home. All you need are almonds, water, and strainer cloth. Another almond substitution is almond flour.

Cauliflower Mash for Mashed Potatoes

Mashed potatoes are one of the biggest forms of comfort food in North America, and can be difficult to give up. It's a big part of family meals, especially holidays like Thanksgiving and Christmas. Mashed cauliflower, which is made pretty much the same way, looks like potatoes, has the same texture of potatoes, and even tastes the same. You can add whatever spices to it that you like, and butter or cheese is always a great addition. Yum!

Fathead Crust for Pizza Crust

Missing out on pizza can be a huge bummer for ketogenic dieters. Pizza is awesome. Pizza is delicious. Even bad pizza is good pizza. Unfortunately, it comes with a ton of carbs, and most of them are in the crusts. Fathead crust is a perfect alternative made from almond meal or flour, grated cheese (mozzarella works best), cream cheese, and an egg. This may be a bit time-consuming, but it's so good! And if you're a big pizza fan, well... it's totally worth getting that amazing pizza taste back.

Portobello Mushrooms for Burger Buns

Everybody loves a good burger. It's a staple in many restaurants and bars, and you'll often find a lot of them bragging that they have the best burger in town, the county, or the state. While you can eat many of the ingredients of a burger on the keto diet, you're missing one of the two most critical ingredients: the bun. Some people are OKAY with missing out on the bun, but for others, you just can't have a good burger without the burger bun. Portobello mushrooms are the perfect substitution for buns, with all the softness and consistency as a regular bun, with a punch more flavor. You won't even miss the white bread when you discover this substitute.

Veggie Noodles for Pasta

There are many people out there who have turned to alternative forms of pasta, and veggie pasta is one of them. Zucchini is the best and makes some beautiful, delicious noodles. There are two options for making veggie pasta: using a spiralizer, which might be stocked in a total cooking store, but also can be ordered online, or, if you're not looking to make the investment before you have tried them, you can cut them up very thinly using a knife or a cheese slicer side on your grater. Veggie pasta is not only better for you and has heaps more nutrients in it, but it's also more flavorful and makes you feel so much better after eating it—other than regular pasta which often makes you feel bloated and overstuffed.

Spaghetti Squash for Pasta

Spaghetti squash is not quite the same as the spaghetti, but it's still pretty delicious. There is a tiny hint of sweetness within it that you won't get from regular pasta and it tastes good with tomato sauce. It also comes with its own bowl and is cheap and easy to make.

Kale Chips for Potato Chips

Chips are basically just deep fried vegetables with a variety of spices sprinkled over them, so there is no reason why you can't do this with any other veggies with just an oven. Kale chips are great, mostly because they literally take 20 minutes to make, and you only need kale, salt, and olive oil. You can add a variety of spices as you wish, but just salt works too. All you have to do is remove the stems so you just get the leafy greens, spread them out on a baking tray, drizzle a tiny amount of olive oil (two teaspoons—you need only a little bit or the chips will be soggy, and if you need more add one drop at a time). Massage the oil into the leaves, and put them in the oven at 300 Fahrenheit for seven minutes before flipping them over and putting them in for another seven minutes. Voila! All the deliciousness of chips with none of the carby downsides!

Meal Prep for Beginners

One of the best steps you can take for any new lifestyle is preparing yourself for it. This involves laying out your workout clothing, organizing your bag so you can grab it easily and go to work, having a car ready and waiting for you every morning—anything.

Meal prep is a great way to prepare yourself for a new diet. Not only do you save money and time by knowing how much you're going to eat and having to avoid working through a mountain of dishes every night, but you'll also be able to fight cravings better and avoid the inevitable time when you start to crave something that you shouldn't.

Meal prep can be done in one of two ways: you cook all your meals altogether for the next few days, or you prep the ingredients so you can have variety in your meals. There are downsides and benefits to both, or you can do a combination of both.

Cooking all at once involves you putting all of your meals for the next four to five days in containers, separating them out. This method works great if you want to spend as little time in the kitchen as possible or you have a busy schedule. It can also be really valuable in that you only have to worry about counting macros the one time. You don't have to do the math every single night, but it can be tiresome to eat the same thing over and over again, though, and it can be easy to fall into a ritual of just eating the same meals over and over again. If this isn't something that you feel you can do, consider your other option.

By cooking just the ingredients, you can make a whole bunch of meals over the course of a week, and mix and match to make what you want. You do have to worry about counting the macros, though, again and again, and you might have to do more dishes.

Doing a combination of the two can be valuable as well. You can do all the meals that require more heavy cooking (think stir-fries, soups, casseroles) while all the meals that don't require too much effort can be prepared (think salad dressings, roasted veggies, chicken breasts, burgers).

To-do List

Now that you've got an idea of what you want to eat, and how your first few weeks will look according to the diet, now it's time to go over your kitchen. Hopefully, your kitchen will already have many of the items you will need to get started. It can be a bit of investment, but it's totally worth it.

- *Clear all cupboards out of carbs.* If you live with people who aren't looking into making the keto change, consider having cabinets specifically for your keto foods. If you live alone, or your family is right there with you, donate it to a local homeless shelter, or give it away.

- *Kitchen tools.* You probably already have things like saucepans and knives, but consider buying a scale. If you're looking to lose or gain weight, a scale is very useful. After a bit of time, you'll be able to eye it without too many issues. Also, a body scale can feel really encouraging (but if you don't want to focus on that number, don't focus on that number). For kitchenware, stick with simple, basic, what you need tools, like a few saucepans, one or two frying pans, a set of knives, a good cutting board, some wooden spoons, and a spatula. Make sure you also have the tools to clean your dishes in your kitchen like sponges, scrubbing tools, dish soap, and gloves.

• *Stock up on keto-friendly foods.* You'll definitely want to stock up on things like oils, condiments, frozen veggies, nuts, and meats in the freezer. These things are always good to have, and they're the kind of thing you wouldn't buy every week. Consider a plan for every week that you go through your entire kitchen and make a list of all the things that you need to stock up on.

• *Ketosis testers.* There are three different options for how to test that you're in Ketosis, and there is information about them in Chapter 2. It's up to you to choose which one will work best for you, and they can be a valuable asset to your keto journey.

Now it's time to really get started. The next chapter will guide you through your first week on keto, and help you with the keto flu, one of the big side effects of just starting out, as well as helping you with sugar cravings.

Chapter 6: The Keto Flu

The first few weeks of the keto diet can be rough. There is not only a lot of change to your day-to-day lifestyle (especially if you're someone who eats a high carb diet and you're quite simply just not used to cooking for yourself), it can also feel pretty terrible thanks to the keto flu.

The keto flu is something you'll probably start feeling within the first few days of the diet. You may not feel it at all. Some people manage to smoothly transition from a regular diet to a low-carb diet without any problem whatsoever. You probably won't be one of them. It can feel very similar to the flu, ergo the name "keto flu".

Symptoms include vomiting, nausea, constipation, diarrhea, headaches, irritability, stomach pain, muscle soreness, muscle weakness, sleeping difficulty, sugar cravings, muscle cramps, dizziness, and poor concentration. Typically, the keto diet will last about a week, but symptoms can last up to a month. The worst will probably happen within these seven days. This can often make first-time keto dieters throw in the towel, but you need to push through— at least for the first seven days.

The first day you probably won't feel much. You will start feeling something by the end of it, however, probably in the middle of the night. You will probably have a hard time sleeping and have to pee a lot. The next day you might feel as if you should just stay in bed all day, and this feeling will worsen, then get better, over the course of about a week. When you've reached that final day, which is a great accomplishment, you might feel better, but because it all depends on the person, you might still be feeling the effects.

Why does this happen? Well, think of your body almost like a house. Your house needs renovation. A big one. The wiring and plumbing are bad, your walls are not insulated, the floorboards have holes, and it's just not a good house. The keto diet is now changing out all the floorboards, properly insulating the walls, and fixing the wiring and plumbing. This will take time, and for a while, you might be sleeping in your house without walls. You have to feel worse before you feel better.

You can reduce symptoms, thankfully. Some of these ways include:

  • *Drink a lot of water.* The keto diet will rapidly shed water stores, and replacing these fluids can help you with symptoms such as fatigue, muscle cramping, and especially digestive issues like diarrhea and constipation.

  • *Avoid strenuous exercise.* If you are someone who works out, or plans on implementing a workout routine with your new diet, hold off for the first week or two, or until you feel like the worst of the symptoms have passed. All of your body's energy is going towards remodeling your body, and it must adapt first. Consider very light exercise, like going on walks or trying out yoga.

  • *Replace electrolytes.* As your levels of insulin decrease, your kidneys reduce and shed the number of electrolytes, such as sodium. Replace them with tablets, gel, or packs to be mixed in a drink. Just check the sugar content. They can be bought at local fitness stores or ordered online.

  • *Get lots of sleep.* Sleep is essential if you want to be successful in any part of your life. You need a good amount of sleep. If you have issues sleeping, consider drinking lavender tea, turn off electronics like cell phones and tablets about an hour before bed, or take a bath or shower. The hot water helps relax your muscles and makes you sleepy.

The keto flu can last several weeks, with the first week being the worst. The first week you might find yourself wanting to quit, but do your best to just push through it. You got this. You're totally up for it.

Don't forget to celebrate when you've reached that seventh week— and not with food. Consider letting yourself do something you've wanted to do for a while, like going to see a movie that you've wanted to see or splurging on concert tickets. Something that will get you up and moving and away from food is your best bet.

Sugar Cravings

Sugar cravings, or carb cravings, are a very common side effect of the keto diet. This isn't just the keto flu; even people who aren't on keto but who are cutting sugar out of their diet feel these effects.

The biggest issue with sugar is that it's mostly a habit. We're used to doing something, so we do it. We're used to having ice cream after dinner. We're used to letting go over the weekend and eating whatever we like. We're used to eating dessert whenever we're over at a friend's house. We're used to buying a sugary coffee drink on our way to work in the morning. When something is such a part of your routine without even thinking about it, you find yourself more used to the habit. You're not just craving the sugar; you're craving the habit.

We've already gone over the bad effects of sugar, but that's not enough. People still smoke cigarettes decades after it was proven just how terrible they are for you. Why? Because it's a habit, and something they're used to doing. You can know all the bad effects of sugar. You could have them be the lock screen of your phone, have them tattooed on the back of your hand, you name it, and yet you might still find yourself craving that candy bar. While, yes, you're craving the dopamine rush in your brain, you're also just used to the idea of going to eat that candy bar.

Now it's time to learn how to deal with it.

The best course of action when it comes to breaking a bad habit is to replace it with a better habit. Buy tea instead of hot chocolate. Reach for the salad rather than the French fries. It can be difficult to fight this impulse, especially if you're so used to giving in. These urges can be pretty powerful, and there is nobody here saying otherwise, or saying that you're bad for giving in to them. It's human nature to stick to the things we're used to, and we're comfortable with, and you're not a failure for feeling these urges. Here are some ideas of what to do when you get the urge for chocolate:

> • *Eat protein.* Protein can help reduce sugar cravings and make you feel full. Even just a handful of nuts could really help. Just make sure not to overindulge and eat too many. They're pretty high in calories, and too much protein in your diet will convert to glucose.

> • *Go for a walk instead.* Walking or any light exercise will help bring dopamine to the brain and reduce the cravings. Just take a spin around the block in the fresh air, and the sun will not only kick that craving to the curb, but it will also put you in a great mood.

> • *Tell yourself, "Later."* By telling yourself this, you'll have something to look forward to. Put off getting sugar the same way you put off getting out of bed or doing the work that you know is due in two days.

> • *Work your way down.* Many people want to jump right into the keto diet and think they can just sustain depriving themselves all at once. Consider working your way down from your sugar level, one step at a time, rather than cutting everything out at once. This will help you feel less deprived,

and you won't find yourself feeling like you're missing out. You could start first by cutting out soda, then processed sugars like what is in candy, then replacing them with other ideas. You could replace soda with water, a handful of candy with berries, a sweet coffee with bulletproof coffee. The choice is yours.

It will also be really, really helpful to identify your triggers early on. Are your triggers social? Do they occur walking past a certain gas station or grocery store? Are they at a certain time of day? Is it something you just do without thinking?

Identify your triggers, and work to change them. Instead of buying a candy bar at the checkout aisle, call your partner and ask if anything else is needed. Instead of heading to the vending machine for that two PM sugar crash, bring a snack from home.

Remember: the craving is temporary. And the pain that comes with it is temporary. However, the feelings of pride and awesomeness will stay with you forever. Plus, you know it's good for you.

Chapter 7: Exercising

When people picture themselves making better life choices, they often picture themselves eating better and then following this up with a lot of cardio and sit-ups. This, of course, can be a part of the ketogenic diet, but first, you need to change many of the ideas you probably have over exercise and dieting.

When the image of someone "dieting" springs to a person's mind, they often think of someone who is eating much less than average and following up this pitiful meal by working out for an hour. This model is not only unsustainable but ridiculous. We've already covered that the keto diet can be full of rich, enjoyable meals that will fuel your body and make you feel good. Exercise can be equally enriching.

Just in case you don't know, exercise is primarily fueled by glucose. When glucose is stored as glycogen, it is the glycogen stores that get burned when you do strenuous exercise. So, you may be wondering how exercising works on the keto diet, considering that you're switching your body over to burning fat.

Some people may read the fact that exercise burns glucose and think that exercise is impossible. Or that they shouldn't bother.

To be clear: you can get by without worrying about exercise. The majority of our health comes from what we eat, and as long as you're moving around a lot during the day in the form of walking and standing, you should be fine. Although, exercise does have its health benefits. It helps makes our bones stronger, enhances muscle growth and sustainability, and is good for the heart. So, implementing even just a light exercise routine is very beneficial.

There are four kinds of exercise you can do:

Aerobic: this is what is commonly known as cardio and is anything that's high intensity and lasts for over three minutes. It predominantly uses carbs as an energy source.

Anaerobic Exercise: this is what people consider interval training. It requires shorter bursts of energy, and carbs are once again its primary source of energy. Think of weight training or high cardio interval training.

Flexibility: this is anything that stretches your body. Think yoga, or after workout stretches. This kind of exercise is great for your joints, improving your muscle range of motion, and helps prevent injuries.

Stability: think balancing exercises and core training. It improves alignment, strengthens muscles, and helps control movements.

What energy is burned really depends on the intensity of your workout, but the gist of it is this:

Low-intensity: fat is used as energy

High-intensity: glycogen is used as energy

Pretty simple, right?

However, that does mean that you need to consume more carbs if you do more high-intensity workouts. It goes back to the fact that the more you work out, the more carbs you need. You're going to have to adjust the carbs based on your lifestyle.

If you exercise more than three times a week, consider looking into a different kind of ketogenic diet, specifically the Targeted Keto Diet.

We already talked a bit about it before, but the idea is that you eat all your carbs around the time you work out. Eat 15 g to 30 g of carbs right before and right after. This gives your muscles glycogen to help your muscles recover, and any extra glucose will be burned away by the workout.

For the first few weeks of the keto diet, exercise will be pretty hard on your body. This means that for this time, you're going to have to take it easy, like with walks and light yoga. The longer your body gets used to burning fats for energy, the better you will feel. You will find your exercise performance will increase after a few weeks.

In the beginning, focus on the diet first, rather than the exercise. Feeding your body with the proper nutrients it needs and letting it adapt to the different fuel source is more important, at first. After your body gets adjusted, you will find it much easier.

Chapter 8: Socializing

You can control your diet in the kitchen, but in other kitchens, not so much. Eating is an essential part of our social life. We have food at parties, when we go out with friends, at the movies, and there aren't very many social settings that don't call for a drink at the end of the night. Unfortunately, when you're on a restrictive diet, keto or otherwise, you find yourself very limited by your options of what you can eat. Not only that, but you're surrounded by temptation wherever you go.

However, you need to socialize and see your friends. That's just how humans work. We need to spend at least some of our time surrounded by people we love and who love us. We need to have mental stimulation from good conversation, laugh at our friend's jokes, and have some good-quality fun with the people in our lives. Even if you're introverted and claim to hate people, you would probably find yourself driven completely stir crazy if you went without talking to anyone real for a few weeks. We're social creatures to our core.

So, how do you get around this? Well, one option would be to just nix any involvement with your friends involving food. This will likely not work because food shapes our social lives. You and a lot of the people you consider close friends probably have the same tastes in restaurants you enjoy going to. The second option would be to take some of the advice you're about to read seriously.

Eating out in restaurants. As people's diets are becoming more and more varied, restaurants have to follow their lead, or they might find themselves fighting for a big enough customer base to keep them from going bankrupt. This is the big reason why many restaurants have vegan and vegetarian options now, and many of them also have gluten-free and dairy-free menus on request for those who have conditions that prohibit them from eating these foods. Whether or not a keto diet menu will join the list in the future, follow these tips until that blessed day finally dawns upon us:

> 1. *Tell your friends about your dietary needs beforehand.* It's like this: if you were completely gluten intolerant, like to the point where you could not eat gluten, you'd die if you did, you'd tell a friend that if you were going out to dinner with them, or if they were making you a meal. By telling your friends upfront about what you can and cannot eat, you can pick a restaurant together. If you want to make the process smoother, research the restaurants with keto-friendly options in the area. Having a list on hand in the note app on your phone will be especially useful for these times rather than you having to go through the local menus each time.

> 2. *Eliminate starch.* If the meal has large amounts of starch as a side dish, like potatoes, rice, or bread, the vast majority of restaurants have salads and roasted or tossed veggies as other options. If it's not listed on the menu, ask! Many restaurants, especially Italian and Mediterranean ones, have bread baskets in the middle; ask for it to be removed. If the meal comes with starch that you did not expect, eliminate it by either throwing it away or offering it to a friend. You can tell the restaurant you have dietary needs beforehand, and this will make the process easier for you.

3. *Add your own healthy fats*. Restaurant food is usually heavy on the carbs and the unhealthy fats, but rarely on the healthy fats. This, of course, depends on the restaurant, but this is a huge chunk of them. Add your own healthy fats by asking for extra butter and drizzling it over your meal. You can ask for olive oil and vinegar salad dressings and use them on a salad. A lot of restaurants prefer the more affordable canola oil, which is far less healthy than olive oil. Seasoned ketogenic dieters know they should always carry a tiny vial of olive oil somewhere on their person.

4. *Ask*. Restaurants should always be completely transparent about what they're putting in their food. They should have no problem answering whatever questions you might have, and if you request to see an ingredient list, that is your right. You have a right to know what is going into your body. Period. If they do seem to have an issue with you looking into their food, or behave like you're crazy, well, you can cross that restaurant off your list of places to go to.

5. *Eat a snack beforehand*. This is especially beneficial if you have a hard time resisting temptation when it's right in front of you, or if you plan to be out for a while. Keep a snack in your bag if you're going out and about with friends. This will help you to stop reaching for the French fries. Just a small bag of nuts and you'll be golden.

6. *Go easy on the alcohol*. While some alcohol is totally OKAY when you're going keto, others are not. Also, be honest. Once in your life you've probably got drunk and eaten your way through an entire pizza or a huge bag of Oreos (no judgment, we've all been there). Getting drunk can lead to you being much less careful about what you're putting in your body. Be careful.

7. *Choose drinks with care.* Water, sparkling water, coffee, tea—these can all be drunk without worry. There are also

many carb friendly alcohol options. It may take some getting used to, but you'll get there.

8. *Keep an eye on sauces.* Sauces often have huge amounts of carbs and sugar in them, especially those that are served in restaurants. Remember: restaurants want you to come again, and they want you to enjoy their food. This often means that they pack a ton of carbs and sugar into it to make it as delicious as possible. This includes sauces. Safe bets usually include vinaigrette, mayo, and hollandaise sauce, but ask for an ingredient list if you're unsure.

9. *Rethink dessert.* If your friends are all ordering dessert, go for a cup of coffee or tea. Ask if the restaurant can make up a cup of berries drizzled in cream if you really want something sweet.

10. *Know when to cheat.* One small plate of French fries every few months is not going to ruin your diet. Knowing when (and how) to cheat can make the restrictions so much easier, and keep your head on straight. If you're visiting a friend in another city and you're visiting a bakery that claims it has the best chocolate cake in the world, a thin slice will not kill your ketosis—but it may open up the doors to cravings, so be warned.

Alcohol

Weirdly enough, alcohol doesn't have nutrition labels. This is because manufacturers argue that because technically alcohol isn't a food, and you don't drink it for nutritional purposes, this means that they don't need one. This can be frustrating for people wanting to stay inside their calorie range, but they still want to have a good time and drink and dance.

Alcohol is another part of the social experience. People love to drink. If the United States of America couldn't get rid of alcohol completely, it's probably not going to be going anywhere, at least not in our lifetimes. It's your choice whether or not you drink. Don't let anyone tell you otherwise.

On the keto diet, you can drink, just not as much as before, and like almost every other food group, your choices are much more limited. Also, you need less alcohol to get drunk, which is a pretty great benefit. However, be careful. Just assume that your tolerance level has gone down by about half until you're sure. Nobody really knows why this is, but the theory is because the liver is busy at work producing and maintaining ketone levels, and it's too busy to take care of the alcohol. There is less capacity to dilute it from the bloodstream.

Alcohol should be enjoyed in moderation, no matter what diet you're on. However, if you're someone who often drinks, as in one to three times a week, and you're not losing weight, consider cutting back on the drinking. It may very well be the culprit.

All of these drinks you'll be able to find at your local liquor store, and the majority, if not all, will be available at any restaurant with a liquor license:

> • *Wine:* Dry wine can be enjoyed with little impact. In a regular glass of dry wine, there are about .5 grams of sugar, and a tiny amount of carb remains, all of which add up to about two carbs per glass. This amount of wine won't affect your diet much, especially if it's not done on the regular and is instead an occasional treat. Sweeter wine, however, can have upwards to four carbs per glass, while a glass of dessert wine can have five to six.
> • *Beer:* Think of drinking beer similar to drinking liquid bread. Some of them have over 14 carbs in a single, 12-ounce bottle. While there are some light beer options out there, it may be best just to stay clear entirely. However, if you really can't resist, or just want a couple of cold ones for a special

occasion, keep this tip in mind: the darker the beer, the more carbs it has.

• *Hard liquor:* There are no carbs in any hard liquors. Not even vodka, which is made of potatoes. As long as you don't add anything like fruit juice or sugar-laden flavorings, you're good to drink as much as you want. You can also add diet sodas (in moderation, remember) to the drinks.

Here is a list of some drink suggestions, ordered from lowest carb intake to highest.

Drink	# of Carbohydrates
Whiskey	0
Dry Martini	0
Brandy	0
Tequila Shot	0
Vodka and Soda Water	0
Bloody Mary	0
Margarita	8
Cosmopolitan	13
Gin and Tonic	16
White Russian	17

Vodka and Orange Juice	28
Rum and Coke	39

- *Coolers:* You mean alcoholic sugar? You may know these things by another name, such as spirit coolers, cider, hard lemonade, wine coolers, the list goes on and on and on. Either way, these things are all packed with sugar and a whole busload of carbs. You might as well just be drinking sugar, so you're much better off to avoid them like the plague. As time passes, more and more sugar-free ones will enter the market, but until that day comes, stick to other drinks.

- Champagne: Don't worry, when you're celebrating your latest promotion or at a friend's wedding or birthday party, you can still toast and sip on the champagne without worrying about the issue on your diet. One glass contains about one gram of net carbs, so sip leisurely.

Activities to do With Friends (That Don't Involve Eating or Drinking)

Food may be a huge part of our social life, but it doesn't have to make up our entire social life. There are plenty of things you can do with friends and family that don't involve either of these things, and you can have loads of fun and create a bucket load of amazing memories without food being at the center of it all.

Your friends and family should be your biggest supporters, so they should understand that you can't eat at the restaurants you used to go to. Let them know what you want to do, and if they really want to see you, they'll make it work. You don't have to go get coffee and a donut every time you see each other—and maybe your friendship could use a little variety.

1. *Try a new restaurant.* Yes, this list is about things that don't involve eating, but think about it: if you find a restaurant that has keto-friendly recipes, it's near the one you usually go to, and your friend is down to try it, go for it. Finding new food to eat and trying new things is one of the great pleasures of life.

2. *Go for a hike.* There is most likely a few local hiking spots in your area that you have been meaning to do but never have for whatever reason. Do it now, and bring the gang. Just make sure to pack plenty of water and some healthy snacks, like nuts and dried meat, such as beef jerky.

3. *Ride around with some bikes.* If there is a local bike rental place, or you have your own bike that hasn't gotten any attention recently, hop on it and take a spin. It's great exercise, you'll get some fresh air, and you'll see a part of your city that you've never seen before. Get peddling; adventure awaits!

4. *Outdoor movie or concert.* Look into your local listings, or on Facebook (events are often posted there). Ask around to see if any people know anything. There are plenty of free concerts, especially in the summer months.

5. *Visit the zoo or aquarium.* Visiting your local zoo or aquarium can be both an educative and fun experience. You can take silly pictures with the animals and often they do training shows. Grab a whole group of friends and go!

6. *Head to the beach.* Who doesn't love laying around in the sun all day in between beach volleyball and taking dips in the ocean? Plus, you can get in some great calorie burning at the beach, whether it's swimming, playing Frisbee, or even just walking on the sand.

7. *Have a craft night.* Have a night where you all get together and paint, or draw, or learn how to knit. You may all be

terrible at it, and all of the crafts may come out looking awful, but you'll have a lot of fun, and you'll learn together.

8. *Take a class together.* Speaking of learning together, taking a class with a friend is always better than taking one alone. Look at your local rec center for classes for adults they're having, like painting, pottery, writing, or even something like book study or cooking. They may even have a class on keto cooking coming up!

9. *Camping.* If you'd just like to get away for a few days with your friends, away from the temptation of carbs, or even just want a few days away from the craziness and bustle of the city, it can be really valuable to enjoy the stillness of camping. You and your friends can hike, tell silly ghost stories around the campfire, and go on night walks (just be sure to bring a flashlight, and prepare yourself, so you don't attract bears).

10. *Try a fitness class.* If you're also looking to include fitness into your lifestyle and have a friend who's also into working out, find a fitness class that you both would enjoy. Your local rec center, YMCA, or gym will have them.

11. *Watch the sunset or sunrise.* This can go hand in hand with camping or going hiking. Either get up really early in the morning or in the evening and watch the sunrise or sunset with a friend or a group. However, if you live somewhere where it's easy to watch the sunset or sunrise from your place (the roof of your apartment building, perhaps?) consider doing that. If you're blanking on where you can watch it, consider checking out a local community group on Facebook. Most cities have them.

12. *Visit a museum or art gallery.* It never hurts to learn a little bit more about history, your town, your state/province, or your country. Keep an eye on the announcements to see if they have upcoming exhibits. Check out your local art

museum for a touch of culture in your life, and, of course, to look at beautiful paintings.

13. *Host a bonfire.* This may only work if you live outside of a city and have a backyard. And well, a lot of stuff to burn. But if you ever find yourself in one of these positions and want to burn stuff (like we all do at times), just do it.

14. *Host a video game tournament.* Really into gaming? Do you or a friend have a great video game console? Or maybe you just got a new game? Either way, get together and host a tournament. Winner gets to wear the gaming crown for the night!

15. *Host a movie night.* This is a great idea for big movie fans. All you really need to host a movie night in your apartment is a Netflix account (or a cheap Blu-ray or DVD player), and a TV. Snacks are optional. Consider going for themes, like romance, Pixar, or horror.

16. *Have them over for dinner.* This could be a great way to develop more understanding about your diet, and plus, there are few better feelings than making something for your loved ones, especially if it's something you know they'll enjoy.

17. *Visit a park, botanical garden, or wildflower field.* Walking in the park with friends is underrated. Getting out in the fresh air, having a good talk, and looking at the beautiful flowers is a great way to spend a beautiful day.

18. *Play some sports.* Get together to shoot hoops, play soccer, or catch. Even go to the park and toss a Frisbee around.

19. *Check out a comedy club.* Who doesn't love a night of laughing with friends? Keep an eye on the local listings, and the comedians who're coming up. Many comedy clubs post clips on their websites, so you'll get a sense of their humor before you go.

20. *See a movie.* Remember: snacks are totally optional, and unfortunately, most movie snacks aren't very keto friendly. If you must snack while you watch the movie, consider bringing something from home.

21. *Volunteer.* Is there a cause you and a friend feel passionate about? Helping the homeless? Working at an animal shelter? Spending time with the elderly? Either way, volunteering is a great way to spend your time, and you might even meet some new people. You won't have time to think about food. Plus, bonus, you get to feel good about helping people (or animals) all day long, which is a great feeling.

22. *Have a board game night.* This is a great way to spend time with friends. You can have only one game, or several, your choice, and have fun arguing over monopoly.

All in all, you shouldn't let your diet stand in the way of you spending time with the people that you love. Your friends and family should absolutely be your biggest supporters, and when they're not, or they question your decisions, it can be difficult.

The keto diet is still relatively new, and because of this, people often make snap judgments. They hear things like "I don't eat pasta," and they wonder why the heck someone would do that. You might find yourself fending off some comments and advice from people who think they're dietitians or nutritionists and family members who don't understand why you can't eat certain foods you used to love.

The best things to do in these situations are to smile and move on. Remember: many people are insecure about their diet, and they might worry that you'll judge them. Just approach anything that is said negatively about your diet with a "you do you, I do me" approach.

Whatever you do, don't give in. Remember: you're making this journey for a reason, and no matter what that reason is, only you can decide if it's a good enough one. If somebody offers you a piece of cake, and you say no, don't feel bad for saying no, even if it is someone's birthday or a special occasion. It can feel odd being the only one at the table not ordering dessert, but once you see the results, it will all be worth it.

Living With Those Who Aren't into Keto

If you find yourself in a situation where you are living with people who are not into the ketogenic diet, it can be rough. You're trying to partake in this diet, probably experiencing major cravings, and find yourself surrounded by people who are eating all of the foods that you love. You probably won't be able to convince the majority of your housemates to partake in the diet with you, but because we can't all live alone, here are some tips:

- *Tell them your reasons.* Remember: comments from friends and family probably come from a place of genuine concern. When this happens, list out the reasons why you're doing it, show them the science, and ask for their support. They might just be worried that you're not getting the proper amount of nutrition you need.

- *Hide the stuff.* Meaning "don't keep the bad foods in front of you". Keep foods like chips and pasta in a different part of the kitchen, and if you can, avoid cooking with it until you don't crave it anymore. You're more likely to reach for the healthy stuff if it's right in front of you.

- *Replace.* There is an entire list of foods here that you can use to replace some of your favorites, such as zucchini spaghetti for spaghetti, and introduce recipes that you know that your family will love. Try adding things with a keto twist, and focus on finding foods that not only fit into your guidelines, but you also know they'll like.

Cheating on Keto

Cheating on a diet happens. Everyone gets tempted occasionally, especially when everyone else is around you eating treats that the keto diet restricts. It can also be hard to stop eating foods that you love. It only gets harder when you go out to restaurants or parties, and all you really want is French fries or the delicious crab cakes everyone else is chowing down on.

However, cheating can help you get through it. It can keep you on track. Cheating, or treating yourself, as most people would prefer to call it, can help you do the keto diet without feeling totally deprived. The only issue is that people rarely cheat on diets in the right way. They don't go into cheating with a plan. This guide will not only teach you how to resist cheating but also teach you how to do it the right way. It will help you get back on the horse without too much of an issue and not feel the side effects for too long.

Of course, you shouldn't cheat for the wrong reasons. Things such as peer pressure, politeness, impulsivity, and bad planning are all terrible reasons.

Peer pressure is the worst reason to do anything. We all remember our parents telling us, no matter what, don't give in to peer pressure, right? If people treat you different for your dietary preferences or give their unwanted opinions, just ignore them. Remember why you're doing this; for you, not them. However, it also goes the other way. Don't try to pressure the people around you into trying your diet, and don't be judgmental of people who are choosing to eat differently. Everyone has a different relationship with food, so focus on yours.

Politeness is the second worst reason to do something, especially if it's something you don't want to do. Your Aunt Martha will get over it if you don't eat a piece of her special dessert at the family dinner. If your friend Connor keeps pushing this new recipe on you that he found, but you can't eat it, just remind him of your dietary requirements and tell him that you wish you could. If they keep pushing, just make up the excuse that you have stomach or health issues.

Impulsivity is the worst kind of cheating. If being polite and peer pressure are the worst reasons to cheat, impulsivity is the worst kind of cheating. It just isn't satisfying. It's over too soon, and you don't enjoy it. Planned cheating can make you feel empowered, reminding you that you're in control of what you put in your body and no one else. Impulse cheating leads to you feeling bad about yourself and like you're out of control. It will also lead to no portion control if you just let yourself eat without thinking.

Inadequate planning can also lead to wrong cheating, such as being out and about and realizing that you don't have a way to feed yourself, so you have to settle for a McDonald's burger or a gas station hot dog. Not only have you wasted a cheat card, but it can also feel unsatisfying. To help avoid this, keep a low-carb, high-fat snack in your bag, briefcase, or car, such as nuts. Or keep a list of restaurants you know provide low-carb options in your phone.

There are some more wrong reasons to cheat. Cheating actually can help you stick to your diet. It enables you to avoid feeling so deprived and like you're missing out. You also add some variety and flexibility to your diet. There are also special occasions like holidays or the birthdays of close family members or friends (having birthday cake at the office does not count). If you're heading over to your mom's house for Christmas, and she has the most amazing Christmas cookies ever, it won't hurt to have one. You just need to learn to say no after one. You need to learn how to cheat consciously.

Cheating consciously requires planning, but it also requires knowing what you're getting into. There are some adverse effects. You're opening the door to things like hunger cravings, sugar cravings, weight gain, blood sugar spikes, sickness, and generally feeling terrible. Your mood can suffer, your skin may have a breakout if you are prone to acne, and you can become gassy.

There's also the issue that if you do suffer from sugar addiction, which is very much a real thing, you really can't eat sugar. Sometimes only a little bit will send you over the edge. You really need to ask yourself, "Can I stop at just one?" If you're thinking it's silly to fall into a pattern of sugar addiction, think of it this way: you wouldn't ask an alcoholic only to have one drink, would you?

Now, if you do find yourself tempted to cheat, try some of these tactics to cheat in a way that won't mess up your diet:

- *Delay:* If you're at a party and you really want to try something, eat something else first. Load up your plate with any low-carb options they have, or snack on a prepackaged low-carb snack that you brought along with this very thing in mind. If you still want something after this, tell yourself that you can have it later. Yes, you'll have a piece of chocolate, but you'll have it tomorrow, or when you get home. More often than not, by the time that you're home, you'll probably not even want it anymore.

- *Cheat deliberately:* Plan your cheats, and take charge of them. Write down when you're going to cheat. Set clear boundaries on what you can and cannot eat. For example, maybe you really love hot chocolate, and you really just want one. Instead of going for the large, like you normally do, make a rule for yourself that you only get the small one. You'll feel just as satisfied as if you got the large one, and you can really take your time to savor every sip.

- *Minimize the damage:* Take only small amounts of whatever you're craving. This goes back to ordering the large instead of the small. If you're out with friends, ask if somebody wants to split a chocolate cake with you instead of someone getting the whole thing, or ask for a bite of theirs. Sometimes just a small bite can really satisfy these cravings.

- *Pick something not high on carbs:* Make a good choice. There are many low-carb keto desserts out there that can be eaten in small portions. Even so, check out the nutritional labels on some of your favorites and find the one with the lower carb count.

- *Cheat after your meal:* Eating fat and protein slows down glucose adsorptions, and will reduce the intensity of your blood sugar spike. It will also help reduce your cravings. You might just be hungry after all.

- *Cheat late:* Cheat after dinner. This limits the window in which your body will go out of low-carb mode, and you will go back into Ketosis overnight. Your body will be burning fat for the rest of the day.

- *Pick something with less sugar:* The ketogenic diet ends up changing your taste buds, as they become more adjusted to eating more whole and healthy foods rather than processed ones. You'll often find that things like candy might taste too sweet. Go for cheats like dark chocolate and low-sugar yogurt.

- *Cheat with fat:* If you're going to cheat on a high-fat diet, make sure you're getting some healthy fats with these cheats. Add butter to bread, fat-rich cream to peaches, and cheese to crackers. You'll find yourself needing fewer carbs to feel satisfied.

- *Cheat with food that matters to you:* Choose foods that you really look forward to having. Like a special family recipe, or if you're in a certain part of town and your favorite bakery is nearby.

- *Cheat before or after workouts:* Cheating right before a workout means that the glucose will be burned off quick, and thus your body will stay in fat burning mode. Cheating after a workout means that you've just burned off whatever glycogen stores you had. This means that whatever carbs you'll consume will be put back into the glycogen stores, rather than converted to fat. This will help prevent your body from being kicked out of Ketosis.

Getting Back on Track

The most important thing to do after you cheat is to get yourself back on track. This is one of the big reasons why the smart thing to do is to plan your cheats carefully and prepare yourself for the aftermath.

Anticipating Hunger Cravings: be prepared for the fact that after you have a plate of pasta, you might want more. If you anticipate this in advance, you can learn from it and stop yourself from reaching for more.

Learn From Them: keep track of your cheats, and figure out what sets you off and learn from it. You can keep a notebook and write the cheats down, as well as how you feel, what triggers them, and what they bring on in you later.

Forgive Yourself: if you do fall off the wagon, it's OKAY. Yes, it happened, but it's also a learning experience. You can always climb back up from this, and tomorrow is always a new day. It's OKAY. Just keep going. You got this.

Chapter 9: You and Keto

Any big lifestyle change, especially one involving your diet, can be rough. Diet is a big part of our life. We've been eating literally since the day we were born, and we've been doing it every day since.

Why do you want to do the keto diet? That is the first question you need to ask yourself. Do you want to lose weight? Feel less stress? Take control of your health and food intake? Want to have more energy? Whatever it is, this can often drag on. Having a good reason is all well and good at the beginning, but getting yourself in good habits to help you along the way is never a bad thing.

To help yourself get through this diet, here are some useful habits to have to help you tackle these moments where your motivation falters a bit:

Don't call it a diet: This book may be labeled the "keto diet" but don't call it that. It's more like the keto lifestyle, not the diet. While many people consider the keto diet something you can jump on and off without thinking about it too much, this won't work to keep the weight off. If you go straight back to eating the way you were before, you'll just end up right back where you started. Don't consider this something temporary that will last only a year. This is going to be a lifestyle change that will likely follow you for multiple years.

Get a glass of water: We often confuse thirst with hunger. This means that when we're thirsty, we reach for food thinking it will satisfy us. What we really need is water. To drink more water, keep the water in front of you. For example, when you work, put the water bottle on your desk.

Measure your progress: Once a week or month, pull out the measuring tape, grab the scale, and write the new numbers down. Keeping track of your progress will help you stay focused and see how far you've come. Keep in mind that while you'll lose a lot of weight during the first few weeks, afterward, you might find you lose about one pound a week. This is completely normal. If you want to measure by measuring tape, about one inch off your waistline equals to about five pounds of body fat. You could also consider keeping a photo diary, where you photograph yourself topless in the mirror about once or twice a month. Apps like MyFitnessPal will help tremendously.

Get enough sleep: Sleep will help you make better choices. Getting better sleep will stop the stress from affecting your day-to-day judgments and generally make your life better. Lack of sleep also stimulates your appetite, meaning you'll want more food than normal. You won't feel satisfied, and you'll just want to keep eating. Take the time to really get the best sleep, and take a break from the alarm clock once or twice a week.

Pick a Mantra: Did you know that negative thinking changes the chemistry of your brain, and negative thinking attracts more negative thinking? Well, good news: positive thinking does the same thing. People really underestimate the power of positive thinking. Picking a mantra, something like "eat to nourish your body" or "90% kitchen, 10% workout" can help you reach your goals. Repeat it to yourself when you particularly feel down or like you're missing out. Pick one you feel suits your lifestyle the best. Here are some ideas:

- *"Progress not perfection."* If you find yourself feeling like you're not doing everything right, say this to yourself to remember that it's okay not to do everything perfectly the first try. It's also important to remember what works for you rather than what works on everyone else. Focus on what works for you.

- *"Color your plate."* This is a great reminder to fill your plate with lots of colorful vegetables and other healthy foods.

- *"Quality and quantity."* It's not just quality; it's also about how much you eat. Healthy food still has calories, and these calories still add up over time. If you have an issue with overeating, say this to yourself every single time you want to eat more, but you're not hungry.

- *"Every day is new."* If you have a hard time forgiving yourself after a slip-up, this uplifting quote is for you. Reminding yourself that you can always begin again tomorrow is a great way to look at things.

Be Persistent

You need to keep going, even when it feels as if there is no progress being made. Plateaus occur after a while. Real change really only comes with consistency. Real, slow-burning consistency. It can take a while to see real change, but when it does happen, it's pretty incredible.

Stay Motivated

Staying motivated, especially when things like plateaus occur, is very hard. Hitting a plateau sometimes seems akin to hitting a rock wall.

Find a cheering squad: having a social circle who are supportive can be groundbreaking. Not only can they keep you on track, but they can remind you how far you've come, and encourage you. Posting about your journey on social media is a great way to do this. Finding people who are also participating in the keto diet is a great find—

mostly thanks to the fact that they'll be able to help you through the rougher parts of the diet. Social media is an incredible thing that enables you to connect with hundreds of millions of people overnight, many of whom are struggling with the same thing. Check out a Facebook group, or the tags on Instagram. Just remember to ignore trolls, vicious internet commenters with nothing nice to say.

Nothing happens overnight: There might be some big changes overnight during the first week, but the likelihood of this keeping up at the same pace is extremely low. Don't be impatient. You might not notice results for nearly six weeks after the initial week.

Keep your goals in minds: Keep them written down somewhere, so you always know where they are and what they are. If you're shopping at the grocery store, keep a little memo in your wallet reminding you why you're heading for the veggies rather than the candy. Keep a list on your fridge of all the reasons you're doing this. Write a list of accomplishments you want to hit, and then as you hit them, tick them off—anything to keep you going.

Make Small Changes

Small habits change everything. Things like drinking more water and learning about nutrition are never something too late to do. And it would be nice if we could just jump into the keto diet without having to worry about completely changing your eating style. However, you might find yourself in way over your head, and all you want to do is eat a giant plate of French fries.

Cutting out foods you love can be tough. There is no shame in taking it easy, at first, and making small changes. This can be anywhere in your journey to a better you—things like taking a nice walk at lunch instead of eating at your desk, and reaching for the veggies and guacamole instead of the regular bag of chips for a snack.

Making small changes benefits you over time because you're turning them into habits. You're replacing the bad habits with the good ones, and instead of depriving yourself, you're whittling them down. Some people out there have gone completely cold turkey, and that works for them, but that might not be for you. You might find yourself relapsing and craving carbs and junk more than ever—not because you want to eat it, but because your body is so dependent on it. Consider just cutting down on your habits, and replacing what's in your fridge with the food you want to eat.

Don't Use Food as Rewards

Rewards specifically imply that you've done something amazing, so why would you choose something that could set you back on your journey? A reward should add to your journey, not make it worse.

What's the point of eating healthy for a week if you just plan on bingeing for a single day by eating whatever you want? Not only will you gain back all the weight you have lost, but you'll also knock yourself right back out of Ketosis, and make the cravings for carbs and sugars worst.

Remember: that sundae you've been thinking about, or the big pizza slice you've been eyeing, will throw you out of Ketosis, rather than being rewarding to you. It will only set you back, moving you right back to first base. Also, thinking of food as rewards can negatively affect your relationship with food by sending you the message that it's only something to be enjoyed on occasion.

Control Emotional Eating

We have all been there. We're bored, tired, stressed, and anxious; you name it, and we end up reaching for the foods that are not good for us. Things like our day-to-day lives can make us feel anxious and alone, and we often reach for food as a way to comfort ourselves. We also reach for food when we have nothing better to do. This needs to stop, not only because it will mess up our macro counting, but it's also not good for us.

Consider these helpful tips:

When stressed: soak in a bath, read a good book, meditate, or do some yoga. Find a healthier way to relax than chowing down.

Low on energy: Your first thought might be to pick up a snack, but if that's not doing it for you, take a walk around the block, listen to some energizing music, or take a short nap. Don't just mindlessly reach for more food—it's likely not the problem.

Lonely or bored: Call a friend and chat for a bit. Take your dog for a walk. Read a book or watch your favorite show on Netflix. Just keep your mind occupied.

Practice Mindful Eating

Mindful eating is when you're just paying attention to your food. You're doing nothing else except eating. This means the following:

- *No distractions.* This means no reading, no watching TV, no driving. This kind of mindless eating will only lead to overeating.

- *Pay attention.* Pay attention to your food. You should; you put a lot of effort into making it. If your mind wanders, keep your attention on your food. Think of it almost like a date that you have to impress.

- *Eat slowly.* It takes time for the signal to reach your brain that you're full. Politeness may have drilled into us that we have to eat everything on our plates, but don't feel too bad. It just means you have leftovers for later!

All in all, that's it! If you follow these healthy tips, you'll be burning those ketones in no time at all!

Conclusion

Congratulations on making it through to the end of *Keto Diet: How to Use the Ketogenic Diet to Lose Weight, Burn Fat, and Increase Mental Clarity, Including How to Get into Ketosis and Fasting on Keto for Beginners*. It should have been informative and provided you with all of the tools you need to achieve your goals, whatever they might be. They can be weight loss, being more focused, building a better life—whatever! You should be able to walk away from reading this knowing where you need to go and that you learned a lot about the keto diet.

The next step is to start the keto diet and keep going. It may be rough for the first few weeks, but it will get better. Track your goals, keep yourself motivated, and really embrace the idea of being a better and healthier you. Your body will be thanking you for years to come, and you'll feel so much better for it.

Remember: you are in control of your diet. You control whether or not you say no to foods that you know are bad for you. You are in control of what foods you stock in your kitchen, what foods you order at a restaurant, how much you eat—everything. You control what goes into your mouth, and you have a right to know what it is doing to your body.

Finally, if you found this book useful in any way, a review on Amazon is always appreciated!

Here's another book by Elizabeth Moore that you might be interested in

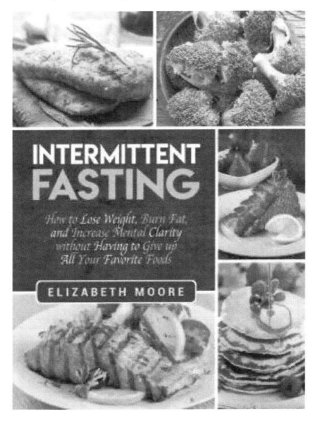

Click here to check out this book!

Printed in Great Britain
by Amazon